TYPOLOGY IN HOMOEOPATHY

Typology in Homoeopathy

Léon Vannier
MD

Translated from *La Typologie et Ses Applications Thérapeutiques: Les Tempéraments, Prototypes et Métatypes* by
Marianne Harling, BM, BCh, FFHom

BEACONSFIELD PUBLISHERS LTD
Beaconsfield, Bucks, England

First published in English 1992

The Types depicted in this book are so universally recognizable that it is often incorrectly assumed that they are based on known people, of whom the drawings are a synthetic reproduction. The author affirms that none of these portraits can be identified with living persons, and that any resemblances to living persons are unintentional and purely coincidental.

French edition © Doin Editeurs 1955, 1976

This translation © Marianne Harling 1992

British Library Cataloguing in Publication Data
Vannier, Léon
  Typology in Homoeopathy. – (The Beaconsfield Homoeopathic Library; no. 13)
  I. Title   II. Series
  615.5

ISBN 0–906584–30–2

Phototypeset by Gem Graphics, Trenance, Mawgan Porth, Cornwall
in 9½ on 12 point Times.
Printed in Great Britain at The Bath Press, Avon.

Translator's Preface

Typology, the classification of human beings according to their physical and psychological characteristics, is as old as medicine itself. It is particularly relevant to those forms of therapy which take account of the whole person, such as homoeopathy.

Dr Léon Vannier, doyen of French homoeopathy in the first half of the twentieth century, founder of the Centre Homéopathique de France and author of many books, including a substantial materia medica, attached great importance to the study of human typology. He believed that it could help the doctor to know his patient better, and the patient to know himself better; and that in homoeopathy the physician had a means of improving the patient's mental and physical well-being, avoiding disorders to which he was constitutionally and temperamentally predisposed, and allowing him to fulfil his natural potential.

Léon Vannier's work on the three calcareous constitutions first described by Nebel – Carbonic, Phosphoric and Fluoric – is well-known. Modified by subsequent writers, it remains an important foundation to the practice of homoeopathy in France today. 'The Constitution is that which is; the Temperament is that which becomes.' The Constitution is fixed, a legacy from the past which must be lived with. Dr Vannier realised that there was another aspect to the human being – his potential which could develop for good or evil. This he called the Temperament. He set himself to determine what different temperaments there were, and how they could be discerned, advised and treated.

Influenced by the work of Dr Henri Favre and his daughter Mme Bessonet-Favre, he took as models for the different human temperaments those Greco-Roman divinities whose names had been attached to the seven heavenly bodies: Apollo (Sun), Luna, Mercury, Venus, Mars, Jupiter, Saturn; and added, as eighth, the Earth, Terra (which was not regarded as a planet in Roman times, although Gaia is included among the Titans). These planetary beings are considered as prototypes of human psycho-physio-pathological behaviour, and each is described at length under the following headings: Morphology (static and kinetic), Intellect, Character, with male and female variations, Changes which occur with age, Diseases to which they are prone, and finally, the Homoeopathic Remedies to which they respond best – usually a group of six to eight related remedies dominated by a major polychrest.

Dr Vannier makes it clear that no human being is a pure prototype, exhibiting a single temperament, and his view is that two, three or even four temperaments will be found in any one person, together or in succession. After the prototypes he describes a number of meta-types – mixed temperaments, which he names after other Olympians not included in the original eight. These are not depicted in such detail as the prototypes, and no remedies are prescribed for them individually. They have been included as an example, an invitation to future typologists to create their own pantheons from among their patients. It could be argued that all the temperaments exist, actually or potentially, in every human being, and that those which are not discerned are important for the very reason of their invisibility.

Some of his critics have accused Dr Vannier of mixing homoeopathy with occultism, but this

v

is not an astrological treatise. There is no mention of birth-dates and no fortunes are told, although physicians are encouraged to warn their patients against defects of health and character to which they may be temperamentally at risk.

This author is a fairly liberal raconteur of Greco-Roman mythology. The gods are tailored to fit his patients, who spring to vivid life, and can be recognised from their similarity to our own experience. This is intensified by the many illustrations – some photographs of statues and pictures from classical until contemporary times, others line drawings by an artist, Robert Simon, who must have been completely at one with Dr Vannier about the appearance of his subjects. As could be expected, most of the historical examples of temperamental types, and most of the literary references, are French. But a reader of any nationality should have no difficulty in finding models nearer home.

M.E.H.

Contents

	Translator's Preface	v
	Foreword	ix
1	Knowledge of the Human Being	1
2	Tradition	5
3	Typological Observation	9

PROTOTYPES

4	Mars	15
5	Saturn	32
6	Apollo	50
7	Venus	70
8	Jupiter	88
9	Mercury	105
10	Luna	120
11	Terra	134

METATYPES

12	Minerva	146
13	Pallas	148
14	Pluto	149
15	Proserpina	151
16	Neptune	152
17	Hebe	154
18	Hercules	155
19	Juno	156
20	Vulcan	158
21	Diana	160
22	Bacchus	162
23	Silenus	164
24	Pan	165
25	Earth Types	166
	Flora	166
	Rhea	167
	Vesta	168
	Ceres	168
	Pomona	169
	Cybele	169
26	Reflections	170
27	Conclusion	174
	Bibliography	175
	Index of Remedies	176

Foreword

The elements which make up this work have been drawn from many sources, old and new. Nothing has been invented; the major concern has been to set out as clearly as possible the results of research and observation.

Each Type presents a number of signs which belong to him or her alone, and these are presented in the following order: first, the dominant characteristics, followed by a general description; then the good and bad qualities inherent in the mind and character of the subject, together with the changes which may take place under influences of a moral or morbid nature; finally a therapy is suggested which could lead to profound modification of the physical and mental condition – indications for the homoeopathic remedies appropriate to the particular circumstances.

In this work, which has taken over thirty-five years to prepare, great help was forthcoming both at the beginning and at the end. In 1906 I had the privilege of knowing Dr Henri Favre, the 'white apostle', as his friends called him. He had a mind whose universality was at first disconcerting, but whose sudden illuminations threw a brilliant clarity upon facts and ideas. He was the author of many works, beginning with the *Série Naturelle Humaine* written during his detention in St. Pélagie Prison, where he spent two years as a political prisoner under the Empire. Then came *Bataille du Ciel* (War in Heaven), a study of the Bible from a political angle, as well as numerous articles which served to arouse and direct the interest of his contemporaries. He died in 1910. I have worked a great deal with his daughter, Madame Bessonet-Favre, who, as a member of the Society of Diplomatic History has also left interesting

works: *Jeanne d'Arc*, *Egide* and lastly, *Typologie*, which appeared in 1906. In this book she expressed general ideas whose truth had not yet been recognised. She died in 1920. I owe to Dr Henri Favre and his daughter an infinite debt for the advice they lavished upon me at the start of my medical career, and for the perceptions they so willingly shared with me. If today I am able to present a fairly complete typological study – a practical therapy which is logical and reasonable, and gets good results – I must admit that my main observations still belong to them.

Everything that had been written on the subject has been studied. Repetition is frequent, since it is difficult to show originality in the definition of a Type – the characteristic signs are as invariant as those of a remedy or a disease. It was necessary to delineate the human function of each Type, so as to give the reader an exact notion of its potentiality. It is hoped that this knowledge will provide him with the elements necessary to guide his direction and outlook, and perhaps also allow him to be more indulgent in his judgement of his contemporaries.

The text of this work had been written for a long time, but I delayed publication because I was not able to obtain the right illustrations. The characteristics, signs and modalities of each Type were well described, but they had never been exactly pictured. Pictures were needed to facilitate the knowledge and understanding of each Type, and this barrier had not previously been overcome. I had the good fortune to interest in my search an artist whose talent was matched only by his modesty; Robert Simon, who after several years of study and patient observation, produced illustrations that were both symbolic and human.

In each of the chapters devoted to a Type you will find pictures which clearly emphasize the characteristics of that person's physiognomy. The originality of Simon's work lies in the fact that he does not show us *one* Marsian, but *several* Marsians, not *one* characteristic Saturnian, but *several* Saturnians. The illustrations he has produced are therefore a powerful aid to the understanding of the Types, because they are truly human. Thanks to his talent the Types have for the first time been exactly pictured. I am greatly indebted to him.

The human being is manifested in his form and by his actions. The study of form constitutes morphology, a subject in which much systematic research has only resulted in artificial classifications, whilst the essence has been insufficiently shown. The study of human dynamics, the actions of an individual, whether physical, biological, intellectual, psychological or moral, is of considerable breadth. These parameters have not previously been studied together in a single being.

Our knowledge of the human being, a living and moving entity, is imperfect. The individual cannot be defined, or reproduced, because his true self remains for the most part unknown.

Typology, to be understood and well applied, requires a knowledge of the types which constitute a human being, whose individual function is thus revealed to us.

La Jonchère, 31 October 1954

1

Knowledge of the Human Being

Typology is the study of the human Type. A type is, as the word implies, an imprint in relief, the result of an impression which gives to a human being a set of characteristics that are personal to him alone. The interpretation of these characteristics permits an understanding of his behaviour and the human functions with which he is endowed.

Every human creature demonstrates a *natural type* and a *social type*, both of which are more or less in agreement with one another. Society moulds the individual through education, both by the constraints it imposes on him and by the customs it requires him to follow, but it must not be forgotten that our basic actions are dictated by the natural type whose impression we received at birth. Our features and bodily shape constitute signficant symbols which express our true behaviour. Behind the person (*persona* = mask) we must always look for the personality. Behind the apparent, which is shaped by convention, we find the real, which cannot be hidden from us if we know the exact significance of the pattern expressed.

Thus a human being is a being who has been created and endowed. He *is* and he *has*. His being and having represent his static and dynamic qualities. His *becoming* is of interest because it is the future expression of his possible activity.

Every human being has a potential. That which an individual *can* do he *must* do in order to maintain his level. But this potential varies in quality and extent, according to the subject. A human being may be one but his potential is manifold. Thus (in the words used by Charles Nicholle to describe a microbe) one can say that

the Human Being also is a true mosaic of possibilities, the sum of which constitute and characterise his unique function.

These possibilities can be revealed in every individual, since they are, like our homoeopathic remedies, significantly expressed – *expressed by signs*. To study them is not merely to analyse. A synthetic vision of these possibilities must be created in our minds if we wish to understand their interaction within each being, and thus to know the normal function of the subject, and to appreciate the morbid deviations which can be foreseen.

A human being is defined by knowledge of his Constitution and his Temperament.

THE CONSTITUTIONS

It may be helpful to recapitulate the essential features of the Constitutions.

The Constitution is *that which is*. The Temperament is *that which becomes*. The constitution of a subject is recognised by observation of the skeleton, by a study of the body's shape, and especially by looking at the way in which its various parts are put together. These connections vary according to the constitution observed, but they are constant throughout life. As they were at birth, so they will remain until death. No treatment can modify them, no physical culture change them. (There is one important exception: orthodontic treatment given at a suitable age can correct deformities in the mouth of a Fluoric, whose other characteristics, however, remain the same.)

The constitution of a human being does not change. It relates to the heredity of the subject,

1

who from his birth is thus *signed*, or rather *signified*.

The development of a human being follows one of three plans – three Constitutions, which I have named Carbonic, Phosphoric and Fluoric.

Why these names, which at first may seem a little strange? In the course of studying the constitutions, and identifying their sensory functional phenomena and objective signs, I was surprised by the frequent correlation with the characteristics of three important remedies in our materia medica: Calcarea Carbonica, Calcarea Phosphorica, and Calcarea Fluorica.

Between them these three forms, Carbonic, Phosphoric and Fluoric, divide the human species into three distinct types, whose morphological characteristics we shall briefly recall. This will allow us to establish the morbid predispositions of a subject, by defining his heredity.

Carbonic Constitution

The structure of the Carbonic is rigid and straight. His upper and lower rows of teeth are in perfect occlusion. The teeth themselves are very white and the central incisors are almost square. When he is in the upright posture, the forearm projects slightly foreward and the thigh and leg are not exactly aligned, though they show no angular deformity. In forced hyperextension of the upper limb, the forearm still forms a slight angle with the upper arm.

The Carbonic is 'basic' and 'fundamental'. He is resistant and stubborn. His directing principle is order, his reasoning always logical. He likes to establish, to organise, to construct; and in whatever situation he finds himself he shows, to a high degree, a strong sense of responsibility.

Phosphoric Constitution

The Phosphoric is expressive and variable in appearance. His upper and lower rows of teeth are in perfect contact at all points, but the palatine arch is often markedly ogival. His teeth are yellow and long; the transverse diameter of the central incisors is definitely less than their vertical diameter. When he is standing erect, with the upper limb in forced hyperextension, the forearm forms a straight line with the humerus. Thigh and leg are likewise perfectly aligned.

The Phosphoric is 'elegant' and 'shapely', he is fragile and has low resistance. Naturally distinguished, the search for perfection is the dominant concern of his life. Aesthetic considerations rule his spirit and dictate his smallest actions. He loves beauty and seeks to express it.

Fluoric Constitution

The build of the Fluoric is unstable and flexible. His upper and lower rows of teeth do not meet correctly. An undershot jaw is normal in the Fluoric. His forearm forms a reflex angle with the humerus, more evident when the upper limb is put into forced hyperextension. Thigh and leg show an angular deformity, an obtuse angle facing forwards.

The Fluoric is 'unstable' in attitude and 'irregular' in function. Uncertain and irresolute, he takes decisions on the spur of the moment, and his plans, always sudden and unpremeditated, are often contradictory. Gifted with extraordinary mimicry, the variety of his brilliant performances is astonishing.

The Phosphoric comes of tubercular heredity, and mineral insufficiency will make of him a tuberculinic. The Fluoric has a syphilitic heredity, and shows the effects of specific disease transmitted by the generations which have preceded him. The diagnosis of Phosphoric or Fluoric gives exact indications of the heredity of the patient; it also provides important ideas concerning the treatment to be instituted to assure the disappearance of acute or chronic manifestations, whose diagnosis by ordinary clinical or technical methods appears very uncertain. A combination of tubercular and syphilitic heredities gives rise to a mixed constitution: Phosphorico-fluoric or Fluorico-phosphoric, depending on the predominance of one or other of these two toxins.

THE TEMPERAMENT

The Constitution is *that which is*; the Temperament is *that which becomes*. The temperament is a dynamic evolution superimposed upon the static constitution of the subject. It cannot be otherwise. During the life of a human being his constitution does not change, but his temperament alters, either getting better and better, or, thwarted by environment or illness, becoming progressively weaker until the characteristic signs of disease appear, whether physical, biological, mental or psychological.

The temperament is the sum of all the possibilities of the subject – physical, biological, psychological, psychic and dynamic. These possibilities are potentially present from birth. Their development characterises the *becoming* of the individual, their realisation determines his future.

The constitution is the *constant* of a being; the temperament is his *variable*, operating within limits which are strictly determined for each individual. Human beings are not all equally endowed, and the mosaic of possibilities which makes up their temperament has to be known if we wish to guide, direct and treat them. Fortunately the temperament, like the constitution, is exactly indicated by signs which only need to be recorded in order that the subject's total reactions can be predicted at any given time. Knowledge of an individual's temperament enables us to forecast his reactions to climate, surroundings or illness. This study is of the greatest importance to the doctor, who can thus foresee, and consequently prevent, diseases to which the subject may be prone.

The constitution indicates the genus to which an individual belongs. The temperament characterises the individual and distinguishes him from others, including those of the same constitution. It is not constant and immutable, like the constitution; it can be modified by both external and internal factors. The environment can influence the temperament, and the individual can also transform it by his own free will. But the changes which can be brought about, whether by environment or as the result of an act of will, are always necessarily limited. Although the temperament is the variable, it must be understood that a variation can only take place within well-defined limits. For centuries these limits have been studied by philosophers, artists and doctors. They are determined by the factors which make up the temperament.

The Genesis of Temperament

The temperament arises from two elements: (i) that which has been bequeathed from the past – Atavism; and (ii) that which can replace it – the Possible.

Atavism

The human being is subject throughout life to the influence of his parents and ancestors. Without embracing the theory that we frequently go through life without realising that it is not the self which is in command, but an ancestral reminiscence which causes us, temporarily, to react as our parents would have done, we must nevertheless admit the importance of the legacy which has been transmitted to us, the power of this hidden force which marks our whole existence, this force which Paracelsus called the 'seminal entity'.

Our tendencies, often described as instincts, are usually hereditary traits transmitted from generation to generation, from which it is difficult to break free. In his work *Heredo*, Léon Daudet described the interior drama which plays itself out in the mind of a Fluoric, and in *Monde des Images* he indicated equally clearly why we, as instinctive beings, act as we do. The results are morbid impulses which may be repeated through the generations from father to son. These tendencies may be good or bad, they can amount to genius or descend to crime, and they can be pathological, related to deep taints transmitted through heredity.

Alcoholism, syphilis and tuberculosis impregnate the organism profoundly; the resulting physical and mental defects are closely related to them. Melancholia, apathy, delusions and *idées fixes*, obsessions and hallucinations, delirium, mania and dementia are often accompanied by the stigmata of degeneration, deviation and malformation.

The Possible

If a human being has to bear throughout life the burden of the taints bequeathed by his ancestors, and if because of them he develops bad tendencies, man nonetheless possesses something which is his alone – the gift of being able to fashion himself and his life with the aid of experience. This force, which Paracelsus called the 'entity of power', is also our original, personal force – our 'Possible'.

These two entities of Paracelsus, the seminal entity and the entity of power, cannot be separated. We are thus subject to two great forces, one of which is the legacy from our forebears which we must overcome, and against which we have to fight; the other, which characterises us from birth, and whose manifestations, more or less favourable, seek to affirm our personality. The human being will develop better if he knows the direction in which he is going; he will do well to realise the alternatives in himself of which he is vaguely aware. When, groping through life, faltering, falling, picking himself up more or less disillusioned or desperate, he finds the energy to renew his efforts, it is because he is upheld by the latent force within. Well-directed, it leads to self-realisation, equilibrium and happiness; used in the wrong way it can make a bad situation worse, leaving the subject an unbalanced and disappointed person.

Perception of the Temperament

The constitution is seen by an observer, whereas the temperament is perceived. This means that a constitution can be diagnosed and defined by the senses, whilst the determination of a temperament requires reasoning supported by an impression. This word could not be more accurately used; it is in fact an *imprint* that we are called upon to judge. Leonardo da Vinci wrote, 'According to the law of the Most High, the body is the work of the soul. It creates its own covering and hammers it from within outwards, like a goldsmith making a vessel decorated in relief.' Thus, having seen the constitution and perceived the temperament of an individual, we can determine the type to which he belongs.

The initial temperament of a subject can be modified by environment, health or climate; his inner life can also transform it. Whether the struggle is from without inwards, or from within outwards, the pattern which that person adopts will show the result. The dynamic of an individual, as revealed by his attitudes, gestures, and movements, can be modified; external changes indicate a transformation of the temperament, the stages of which may be studied.

However, this tranformation has its limits. These limits apply as much to development, progress and blossoming as they do to repression, which restricts the individual, crippling him in his struggle against environmental factors. It must also be understood that even though an individual can undergo remarkable transformations, his basic temperament remains the same. It is therefore practicable, using one's knowledge of the constitutional factors, to *heal a temperament*, restoring to it an order which it has never known, or which it has abandoned for extrinsic or intrinsic personal factors.

Thus the observation of humanity teaches us important lessons about the aptitudes, general tendencies and heredity of an individual (Constitution), but also permits us to appreciate the particular possibilities belonging to him (Temperament). It does not indicate the fatal, invariable and inevitable destiny of a subject, but rather his possible future, whose variations can be foreseen, directed and guided.

2

Tradition

Typology is not a new science. Complete systems of symbolic types are to be found in the sacred books and mythology of ancient peoples. Each god represents a particular function corresponding to a natural and a social harmony. When the Ancients wished to create images of the gods, their artists took their models from humanity. The gods were made in the images of men – Prototypes – whose proportions and shapes influenced the canons of later art. Only the facial expression was left indeterminate, barely sketched in; thus initiation was respected, and true knowledge guarded. The myth attached to each prototype illustrated in this way allowed some understanding of its functional play. Mythology offers us a veritable textbook of the science of Types, together with a system of comparative psychology.

The Ancients lacked our resources for the collection and dissemination of ideas. Their ingenuity consisted in uniting a group of different phenomena under names and symbols which only the initiated could understand. The same name might apply to a god, a star, a metal, a physical or chemical function, as well as to a social category with its particular mentality and characteristic appearance. The following are examples of these:

Mars: iron, diamond, vulture, pike, wolf, war, gall.

Saturn: lead, onyx, hoopoe, cuttlefish, mole, spleen, incorruptibility.

Jupiter: tin, sapphire, eagle, dolphin, stag, liver, power.

A true understanding of mediaeval thinking requires some knowledge of the contemporary state of mind. A revolution had just taken place among philosophers and sages. In opposition to the pantheism of Aristotle, the Jewish, Christian and Islamic religions had united in declaring to men that God had freely created the world, that He had made man free, giving him a personal and immortal soul which would bear future responsibility for actions taken during life.

The human being gradually emerges as a Being created for a definite purpose, for a destiny which the observer seeks to know – less from a desire to assist in the evolution of the individual than out of intense curiosity. Central to the transports of faith which move him, there is a seed of pride which will grow in the years to come; he has grasped what the common run of mortals do not imagine, he knows how to 'foresee', he dares to 'predict'. The Universe belongs to him, thanks to the Law of Analogy, which holds the key to all mysteries. Macrocosm and Microcosm, great cosmos and small cosmos, big world and little world; double creation in which one reflects the other. *All is in everything, all can be found.*

The religious character of the era encouraged the search for 'signatures'. 'Medicine', wrote Crollius, 'has been divinely illustrated for us in the book of Nature', that is to say, by Heaven and Earth. 'Be sure that it can be known and researched by Chiromancy (palmistry) and Physiognomy.' *All is inscribed, all is signified, all can be known.* The signatures sought for could be divided into two groups – Animal Signatures and Celestial Signatures.

ANIMAL SIGNATURES

The comparison of human beings with animals, easy because it required no intellectual effort, began to arouse the interest of observers. The first known work of this kind is attributed to the sophist Adamanthus. He wrote, 'We find in some people the likeness to birds or animals which portray certain passions. And whilst they may not be perfectly exact nor very pronounced, it is nonetheless true that the face of man can show this likeness. The appearance of animals is never deceptive and always shows what they are like interiorly. Look at the lion; his strength and courage are proclaimed by the fire of his eyes and the vigour of his tensed limbs. The leopard is impetuous and angry, but treacherous, and only attacks when he can take by surprise. He is bold and fearful at the same time; this mixture of cowardice and courage can easily be discerned from his exterior. The bear is wicked, cruel and rascally; the wild boar is violent and sudden in his anger. But take the ox; does he not embody goodness and majesty? See how the horse advances proudly, inviting flattery and admiration. Dishonesty and knavery are illustrated by the fox. The monkey is a tease, and seems born to provoke amusement and laughter. The sheep embodies simplicity; the goat, extravagance; the pig, uncleanliness and gluttony.'

What has just been said is equally true of reptiles and birds. Animal features in a human are something that no able physiognomist should ignore. Yellowish eyes, rather deep-set, recall the gaze of a lion; if they are very deep-set, mistrust what lies behind, it may be a monkey; if they are prominent, think of an ox.

After the sophist Adamanthus came Porta, who, in 1652, in the second volume of his *Pisionomia del Huomo* recites a veritable animal classification of human beings. Not only is the human face compared with the corresponding animal analogue, but his study is extended to include the feet and the hands, which are compared to the paws of animals. Many pictures illustrate Porta's work, showing the relations which exist between certain parts of the human body and corresponding parts of animals.[1]

Thus comparative studies were made of the eyes of the owl, the beak of an eagle (which resembles a curved nose beneath a flat forehead), the gaze of an ox, a dog and a lion, the brow and ears of a donkey, the eyes, nose and lips of a pig, and the general appearance of a monkey, a horse, a bull, a sheep, a goat and a cat. Very curious comparisons were drawn between the hindquarters of animals and the corresponding configurations of the lower limbs of certain men. The tense, spare legs of a greyhound, the rumps of cattle, the claws of birds, the cloven feet of sheep and the hooves of horses were used as standards of comparison for the legs, hands and feet of human beings. But no real conclusions are drawn from these relationships, which become evident as soon as they are pointed out. They cannot simply be dismissed as ridiculous. In the course of examining patients, have you not sometimes met with a woman whose dry, flat, medially concave thighs were covered, like her legs, with abundant hair? By a natural association of ideas, you may have thought of the extremities of a goat, and then of the Satyrs, whose tendency to drunkenness was legendary.

CELESTIAL SIGNATURES

During the Middle Ages it was commonly held that the heavenly bodies had a profound effect upon humans. Some depended upon Mars, others upon Saturn; some were under Jupiter, others under Venus. Thus each person was dominated by a planet, which determined and justified his actions.

Seers sought to establish which astral or planetary influences were directing the life of a human being towards its inevitable destiny. Their methods varied: they might observe the stars in order to learn the future of an individual, and uncover the stages of his progress by casting his horoscope; or they might observe the individual himself, seeking within him the astral signatures. This examination could include the whole person, or just one specific area, such as the face or the hand. Astrology, Physiognomy and Chiromancy were the three procedures used, but the guiding principle remained the same: Macrocosm and Microcosm, as above, so below, *The Law of Analogy dominated creation.*

Nature rejoices in Nature.

Like seeks Like.

Man is a reflection of the universe, and the highest knowledge consists in finding the likeness which unites man to God, by observing the signs expressive of his destiny.

Some very curious works were published, most of them obscure and diffuse, but always containing the same astral nomenclature: Saturn, Mars, Sun, Venus, Jupiter, Mercury, Moon. These are the heavenly bodies which influence human destiny by means of character, faculties, passions and temperament. Whilst allowing for good influences and bad influences, Destiny is represented as wholly deterministic. The human being, subject as he is to mysterious forces from which he cannot free himself, must submit to his destiny without the power to resist it.

Such thinking will at once call forth a reaction in reflective minds who do not wish to see science 'occultised' by the beliefs of false teachers, whose only task would seem to be the prediction of the future in order to condemn their wretched listeners. *'We have the planets in ourselves'*, wrote Paracelsus. 'Certainly it is necessary to explain the Microcosm. Just as the firmament of heaven, with all its constellations and other attributes, exists according to its own laws, so man shall be as powerfully constelled by the stars within him and around him. And just as the sky is supported by its own forces, and is not governed by any other creature, so neither is man's sky governed by other creatures, but exists in itself, a free and powerful firmament which takes orders from no one.'

If man knows his own 'sky', that is to say, the highest he is capable of, his *having* and his *becoming*, then he knows his place in the universe, and how to behave and to evolve. This is what is meant by Paracelsus: 'The wise man rules the stars.' We are a long way from blind fate. The fatalism that would dominate a human being from his birth saddens and shocks those for whom all human action must lead to perfection. Firmly convinced that there is a future life, they ponder with anxiety the account they must render of that which was confided to their care.

'Astra regunt homines, sed regit Deus.' The stars rule men, but God rules (all). God is invoked here, Deus Sabaoth, the God of the stars and of the firmament whose signs allow us better to understand ourselves and others. Thus astrologers – real ones – study in detail the celestial map of each individual, the 'birth-chart' which they construct with great care, noting in the Zodiac the situation of the planets at the time and place of birth. There they find indications for the possible future of each one. We do not say the future is fated, because every destiny can be – to use a mediaeval expression – 'conjured' with. Celestial forces can always be placated.

Sages of a medical calling were enthusiastic. Their status as healers was exalted by the notion that they might be able, by human means, to alter Destiny, conjure with Fate. A whole new therapeutic system appeared, founded upon plants, minerals, and other substances whose qualities had long been studied. Saturnian plants were suitable for Saturnian people, Jupiterian plants for Jupiterians, and so on. From this evolved a real materia medica, founded upon Nature, the use of which depended exclusively upon the Law of Analogy.

'All things are pictured' (Paracelsus). Paracelsus in his writings, Crollius in his *Basilique Chimique* and *Treatise on Signatures*, Helvetius in his *Microscopicum Physiognominae Medicum*, Zahr in his *Liber Admirabilis*, all relate marvellous elements which, even in our time, are the surest guides to the observation of a Type and its modification.

From the point of view of pure study, the

following must also be mentioned: the interesting works of Porta, *Della Fisiognomia Celesta,* (1652), those of Perruchio on the lines of the face and their astral correspondence – an idea taken up by Cardan, who, after publishing his *De la Subtilité*, followed it with a magnificent album, *Metascopie* (1658); those of Agrippa describing the proportions and the influences which govern the life of a human being.

If we bring together the ancient concept of *mythological types* and the mediaeval concept of *planetary types*, we are at once aware that the two classifications complement one another in form and character. The astral language completes the mythical legend. The humanism of the Middle Ages achieves a more precise knowledge of Being than does Antiquity. It is not satisfied by the astrological explanation – it searches for exact pictorial signs which correspond to the future it needs to know and hopes to modify. 'Mythological illustration' and 'astral nomenclature' are expressions of the same vision seen at two different epochs. Belief in planetary influence was not confined to the Middle Ages. It existed from ancient times, well before Greek sculpture. Egypt has yielded up too many inscriptions based on a knowledge of the Zodiac for there to be any remaining doubt on the matter.

The art of the Middle Ages preserved the old tradition. The study of proportion was the constant preoccupation of the artist, but he no longer sought just to catch an attitude or gesture; he wanted to express the thought of the person he was depicting, so he ceased to limit himself to faces and bodies. Albrecht Dürer gave hints as to the different proportions of the Types, but the forerunner of change was that universal genius, Leonardo da Vinci, who brought a mathematical element into observation, and established standards. Later, with deeper knowledge, his interest moved from the Type to the Individual. The Middle Ages was an astonishing period, during which the spirit of man was exalted by mystical enthusiasm. The true Masters, prophetic figures, were distinguished by their ardent humility: Crollius the Sage, Saint Francis of Assisi, Leonardo da Vinci, mathematician and painter, to say nothing of those remarkable builders whose names remain unknown to us but who left us such incomparable churches. Thus the latent energy of the cloister was seized by the mass of the people, who paid their joyful homage to God by raising towards Him the spires of their cathedrals.

3

Typological Observation

The purpose of typological observation is knowledge of the human function, inherent in each being and consisting of the sum of the possibilities of each being. These possibilities, physical, chemical, biological, psychological and dynamic, constitute many potential factors whose right development will give the individual his essential characteristics. A man should be aware of them, and apply himself with all his strength to putting them to work in the right way. Acting thus he is simply fulfilling his function, a duty which was laid on him at birth and which he must discharge. There is good sense in the phrase which has for centuries referred to the dead as *defunct* (from the Latin 'functus', acquitted).

Life is a profound and wonderful mystery, and without wishing to argue about its origins, which we should reverence, we may usefully consider the multiplicity of living organisms, animal and vegetable. Whilst science places all other animals into different groups according to their size, shape, constitution, behaviour, etc., the human being is considered as resembling no one but himself. In portraying the human body an artist may take account of individual characteristics of form and colour, but the physician, whose business it is to examine, observe and treat people, is often unaware of any difference between them. He thinks he knows Man, but knows nothing of the individual man.

PROTOTYPES AND METATYPES

Man sees himself comparatively, as similar or different to others. It is therefore essential to establish for each order of the series a unity of types to which the observer can relate faces and bodily configurations. This is the natural 'gnomon' – the physiognomon or fixed indication of the type as described by Aristotle, Polemon, Adamanthus and Melampode, who made of physiognomy a branch of the natural sciences of medicine and philosophy. Listen to Aristotle: 'Physiognomy is concerned with the passions of the soul and the phenomena which accompany them, as well as with the circumstances which change and transmute the signs.' No animal has been made or created which could inhabit the body and soul of another animal. The further one advances in science, the more one is convinced that each animal being must be considered in its typical form. The first observers began this study in three ways:

1) Some, taking their models from the animal world, attributed to each man a certain animal figure which corresponded to a particular kind of soul.
2) Others distinguished between the different races of men, considering their various customs as signs.
3) Finally, others judged that the facial characteristics associated with certain moral habits occur in individuals showing the same signs, and this enabled them to distinguish and classify psychological types.

Thus we can list three kinds of observation: zoological, ethnological, and psychological. The object of typology is to unite these three kinds of observation in order to synthesize from them the portrait of a human being. Following the astral nomenclature so dear to the Middle Ages, which corresponds exactly to mythological nomenclature, we can describe eight types by the characteristics which each possesses.

These are: Mars, Saturn, Apollo, Jupiter, Venus, Mercury, Luna and Terra. Together they make up a scale analogous to the seven notes of the musical octave, in which the eighth type described, Terra, can be regarded as the minor octave of the first type, Mars. It is important to understand that none of these types is ever met with in a pure state.

The types which we describe are Prototypes, which appeared later, and whose structure is now well established. This knowledge is valuable, since it enables us to look for characteristic signs in the observed subject, and thence to unravel the morphological and psychological complex with which we have been presented.

To quote Aristotle, every human creature shows a number of physiognomons. We shall never be faced with a pure prototype, but we may see several combinations of prototypes. Such a combination is called a Metatype, and our work consists in assigning the subject to his constitutional metatype. Knowing the characteristic indications for each prototype, this task would at first appear to be relatively simple. But we must take account of the mask of social patterns by which the subject is concealed. Behind the person ('persona' = mask) lies the true personality. This is the same problem that the clinician must solve in medicine. Behind the apparent he must find the real, if he does not wish to be deceived in diagnosis and fail in therapy. You will now appreciate the need to study Prototypes, in order to understand the Metatype who stands before you.

The mixture of classes and races, and the proliferation of knowledge and ideas, make it very rare nowadays to find men so simple that their lives are activated by a single function. The human function, as we understand it, presents a complex which it is our duty to clarify in the light of the composite types presented by the individual. By determining his metatype we shall achieve a deeper knowledge of his functional behaviour, whose variability often worries those around him and disconcerts the subject himself, so that he fails to achieve a balance in his life.

The types which constitute his metatype may not agree with one another. They may be incompatible, or, worse still, antagonistic. This results in a dissonance that manifests itself in disorders ranging from simple nervous tension to severe episodes and outbreaks of violence, epileptiform crises, manic depression and feelings of persecution. The patient, seeking in vain for rest, cannot return to his normal state because he does not know what it is, and neither, alas, does his psychiatrist. He remains a stranger to the function for which he was created, and becomes progressively more alienated.

In eras of transformation, when ideas, customs, beliefs and sentiments underwent great change, physiognomies also changed, and attitudes, like faces, became more defined or subtly different. Several generations go to make up an era, and types have been described from the Middle Ages, the Renaissance, the Eighteenth Century, the Revolutionary and the Romantic Periods. A predominant prototype would emerge from the collective signs of an era. Such was Saturn at the time of Henry II and Charles V, Jupiter at the time of Louis XIV, Mercury in our own epoch of agitation and demonstrations. It is an interesting fact that the interior decoration and furnishings of houses also underwent change. The plain furniture of the Renaissance and the sad interiors of the Saturnian period contrast vigorously with the shiny giltwork and colourful tapestries of Jupiterian days. Today everything is subservient to practical use.

At a time when brute instinct and muscular strength was dominant, the body grew at the expense of the head, and a low receding forehead contrasted with an exaggerated occiput. This was the acephalous type of primitive beings and warlike tribes. But when intellectual culture flourishes and the cerebral faculties are dominant, the forehead becomes higher, the occiput smaller, and the head develops at the expense of the body, which tends to be frail and to lose its vigour.

Function

Considering human beings as a whole, we can distinguish three orders of function, the first relating to the independent type, the second to members of the herd, and the third to the 'directed' type.

'In my opinion', wrote Alexander Dumas the Younger, 'there are three or four moulds in which men have been cast by Nature. Most of them take the exact shape of the mould; these are the ordinary folk who make up the herd. But some, with whom Nature has been more prodigal, will stretch the mould, or sometimes even break it; these are superior beings from amongst whom the shepherds are chosen. People can be recognised as belonging to one or other group, from signs which it is impossible to conceal.'[1]

The superior man is the one who develops to the full those gifts which have been given to him. Self-realisation brings him freedom and happiness. But if he wishes to keep his autonomy, to be truly independent, then all his life must be devoted to ascending the ladder towards his Creator, to whom he must bear witness by avoiding the distractions and temptations which beset him. The 'independent' type isolates himself from everything and everyone and may even be unknown to his nearest neighbours. He may give himself to causes; but he does not mix with other people, nor let himself be absorbed by them.

The signs of conformity or independence may be seen in the forehead – low or high, narrow or broad; and in other traits – a manner which is servile or haughty, arrogant or reserved; and most of all in the eyes, those mirrors of the soul whose intimate feelings they reflect so marvellously. An individual who is truly free and independent may not be capable of submitting to a discipline; yet he knows how to handle himself and respect the social order, whilst still following the law of his own evolution. This is true diplomacy, marked by harmony of language, attitude and action.

Members of the human herd are as vulgar as they are common; the type is easily recognised. These individuals have no outstanding physiognomy; the expression on their faces is blank, because they have nothing to express. Their eyes are vague and lustreless, manifesting passivity. Their faces look like everyone else's; see one and you have seen them all. Their features are unremarkable, their attitudes ordinary, the gait heavy. These colourless beings have human faces, but like Panurge's sheep would jump into the abyss if ordered to do so by an unscrupulous leader. Skilfully marshalled, they are the cyphers who lend fictitious value to a clever dictator. In elections they ensure the triumph of mediocrity.

In addition to the independent type and the herd type, Mme Bessonet-Favre adds a 'directed' type, whose functional play she clearly describes. The directed type is that of a man who submits voluntarily to a discipline, understanding the need for social hierarchy and functions. He shows no sign of servility, but it is clear that he obeys without question in order to avoid risks or responsibility. The directed man is not a parasite, and is certainly not a neutral type, but he lacks the audacity and vigour one would find in an independent type. He always belongs to a school, a party, a doctrine or a system that directs his mind, his soul and his actions. He acts and thinks like those who share his opinions. Independent type, herd type and directed type – these constitute the three modes of being of an individual, three functional modes which must be borne in mind when observing the subject.

It is also essential to distinguish the psychology of a man from that of a woman, because it is not possible, using the same standards, to compare the values of two beings so different in so many respects. Their physiology and constitution, their feelings and mentalities, are different. A woman is a sensitive, vibrant creature. Her feelings are the motives for her impulses, desires and actions. In man, sensibility is more muscular and intellectual; born

[1] Alexander Dumas, *New Letter to Junius* (23 Jan. 1871).

from curiosity, it is nourished by emotion and becomes desire. Masculine egotism is very different from feminine egotism. A woman loves herself, a man admires himself. Thus a woman is jealous about her body and her beauty, whereas a man is more concerned about his reputation and his amour-propre. Reason and logic are the masculine qualities. A man sums up, whilst a woman judges with her senses. Some men have feminine sensitivity, some women have masculine intellectuality. In these cases the socialised roles may be reversed. The woman becomes active and authoritarian, the man passive and timid, and in each appear, more or less developed, the qualities of the opposite sex.

Typological diagnosis, in revealing the constitutional make-up of a person, will enable us to describe accurately the human potential of that individual. To conclude: the observer of types is confronted with a human creature to whom he must allot a metatype, by putting together the different signs which correspond to each constitutional prototype. Is there a rule which could foretell the factors which bring some types together more than others? No, although in the course of our study we shall come to know the antipathies and sympathies which exist between prototypes, and learn better the incompatibilities which divide human beings and the points in common which unite them.

One fact is evident: each metatype is usually made up from a combination of three prototypes. We say usually, because there are cases in which only two prototypes are associated, and others, more complicated, involving four prototypes. But three prototypes is the number most often found in the metatype of any observed subject.

Now the metatype bestowed upon a child at birth can be modified. This is not to say that the constitution can change, but that the predominance of one prototype may increase over the years, especially if the individual does not know himself, nor recognise the advantages to be drawn from the three groups of qualities of

which he is the potential inheritor. For instance, a life-span of sixty years can be divided into three periods of twenty years, during each of which a different prototype exerts a dominant influence. In the course of his existence the individual seems to change; in reality he is only replacing one group of qualities and aptitudes that belongs to one prototype by another group belonging to a different prototype, which then becomes predominant.

Finally, some prototypes contradict and oppose one another; the resulting traumas and frustrations upset the subject's equilibrium. The troubles and illnesses which we are called upon to treat are not always infectious or microbial in origin. The patient presents his illness through certain symptoms which are his interpretation of his own reactions; he creates *his* sickness by giving it the form in which it is seen, but in reality the cause lies within himself. More often than not his troubles arise from the conflict which shakes him so violently, a conflict between two essentially incompatible prototypes.

THE TECHNIQUES OF OBSERVATION

Every human being is, to use a mediaeval term, a 'Semnotheus', a 'bearer of signs', which the observer must be able to interpret.

First it is necessary to establish the Constitution of the subject, which will yield information about his heredity and general tendencies. 'It is good', says Aristotle in his *Physiognomy*, 'to have a method of unifying all the signs which are observed in any particular type. This method is useful, not only for picking out the attitudes held in common by beings, but also for distinguishing between the particular characteristics which appear to be similar in several individuals motivated by the same drives.'

In the course of his observation, the typologist, especially if he is a beginner, would do well to follow a standard technique to ensure that nothing is left out, even if this means recording negative signs. We consider in turn the static and dynamic aspects of the subject.

Static

Height

Without resorting to exact anthropometric measurements, we distinguish three types: tall, medium and short.

Tall: Saturn, Mars, Apollo; *Medium:* Jupiter, Venus, Mercury; *Short:* Luna, Terra.

Skull

The shape of the skull admits of two varieties: dolichocephalic (long-headed) and brachy-cephalic (short-headed).

Face

Taken as a whole, the human face comes in five geometrical shapes. These are: square, circle, ellipse, triangle and cone.

Mme Bessonet-Favre produced a useful classification, in which the shape of the human face is compared to eight easily-remembered natural objects corresponding to the eight principal Types. Thus:

Face shaped like	a date	Mars
„ „ „	an almond	Saturn
„ „ „	an olive	Apollo
„ „ „	an acorn	Jupiter
„ „ „	an egg	Venus
„ „ „	a hazelnut	Mercury
„ „ „	a walnut	Luna
„ „ „	a chestnut	Terra

Forehead

The forehead can be vertical, receding or prominent. It can be broad or narrow, smooth or wrinkled. Wrinkles on the forehead are significant.

Ears

These may be long or short, flat or whorled, close to the head or flapping free. The lower lobe can be small or large, hard or soft.

Nose

The nose can be long or short, straight, aquiline with an upper convexity, or retroussé with an upper concavity. The nostrils may be broad or narrow, flared or closed.

Mouth

The mouth is open or shut, wide or narrow. The lips are thin or well-developed. The upper lip usually projects above the lower. When the reverse is the case it is worthy of note.

Chin

The chin can be long and prominent, like a boot (Mars); long and straight like that of a horse (Saturn); short or receding (showing lack of will-power); round or square; or fat and dimpled.

Eyes

The eye is the mirror of the soul, the mysterious lamp which lights up the eternal 'me' of a human being. It is also the mirror of the body, and as a result of the work of Peczely, we are now able to interpret the signs which appear in the iris during the course of a disease.[2] The eye can be clear, luminous, sparkling or scintillating, troubled, dull, dark or cold.

In the eye can be seen the magnetic power of a free person, the servility and passivity of a member of the herd, the rebellious frustration of an independent type.

Eyebrows

They may be horizontal and straight (Terra), or arched like a circumflex accent (Saturn). The closer the eyebrows are to the eyes, the more serious and stable will be the character of that individual. A wider space between eye and brow denotes a light and mobile character.

Body

The relative proportions between body and head must be noted, as well as any harmony, disharmony or asymmetry. The waist may be high or low. The stomach may be flat, rounded or protuberant.

Limbs

The limbs may be long or short, with well or poorly developed muscles, and thin or fat. The

[2] Léon Vannier, *Le Diagnostic de Maladie par les Yeux: Précis d'Iriscopie*, 3rd edn (Doin, 1951).

joints may be prominent or hidden in fat, craggy or plump and dimpled, fine or coarse, dry or oedematous. The hands may be long or short, the fingers square, spatulate or slender.

The feet may be arched, long or short, thin or fat. Remember the Book of Job: 'The Creator put a sign in the hand of every man, so that each should know his own work.' Palmistry is a chapter in the history of typological observation, as are iridology and graphology.

Kinetic

We must consider the subject as he moves, and study his stance, gait, gestures and even his voice, all of which will show different characteristics according to his type.

Stance

The stance depends on the body's balance system. A person cannot stand or sit without maintaining his equilibrium by unconscious compensatory movements of the muscles, allowing him to keep his chosen position. But his stance also varies according to the feelings which animate him, of which each type will give its own interpretation. Thus:

Arrogant and provocative	Mars
Bent and weary	Saturn
Cool and gracious	Apollo
Imposing and Olympian	Jupiter
Indolent and relaxed	Venus
Quick and nervous	Mercury
Restless and whimsical	Luna
Heavy and torpid	Terra

Gait

Gait precedes muscular activity. Balzac wrote, 'Gait is the physiognomy of the body.' It can be:

Mechanical and jerky	Mars
Slow (flat-footed)	Saturn
Gracious and supple	Apollo
Solemn	Jupiter
Lazy	Venus
Gliding and lively	Mercury
Erratic	Luna
Ponderous	Terra

Gestures

Gestures will also reveal the type. These are:

Sudden and frequent	Mars
Rare and awkward	Saturn
Slow and harmonious	Apollo
Measured	Jupiter
Voluminous	Venus
Rapid and neat	Mercury
Incoherent	Luna
Coarse	Terra

By this means you build up a collection of easily observed signs, whose combination provides the material with which to establish a typological diagnosis. Finally, it is evident that typology provides the observer with signs that relate to symptoms in the homoeopathic materia medica. A case may present with so many symptoms that it is impossible to use them all. Amongst them will be found some characteristics which relate only to a single remedy, and others, less defined, which may serve to validate the original impression. The whole art of the homoeopathic practitioner consists in choosing amongst the patient's numerous symptoms those which most truly indicate the simillimum.

Similarly, in typological observation, the observer must evaluate the signs which he has discovered in his subject. Although it is unlikely that he will ever be faced with an absolutely pure type, he will see a mixture of types, and must call upon his wisdom and experience to unravel the complex, deciding which type for the time being is predominant.

Remember that this is a serious matter, and not a question of telling fortunes or reading the stars. Our object is to discover the 'human function' of the subject, to reveal his potentialities, in order to foresee what could become of him and to guide him in his choice of destiny.

PROTOTYPES
4

Mars

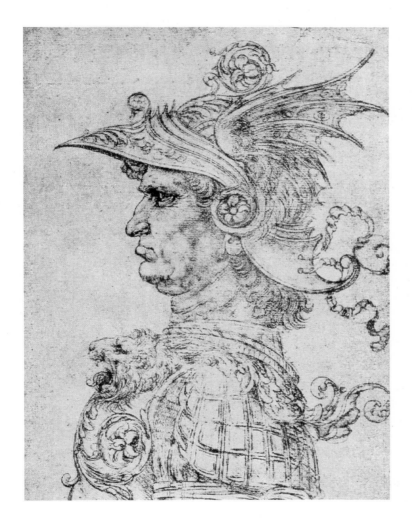

Leonardo da Vinci, *Bust of a Warrior*, (Collection
Malcom: from Gazette des Beaux-Arts)

Mars is Juno's son, but is drier and harder than she is. True to his origins, he is influenced by the iron and fire from which he forged his first weapons.

More successful than Vulcan, his lame brother, it is easy for him to steal the latter's seductive wife, Venus. The Romans, who honoured him above all the gods, called him 'Gradus', the one who takes big steps. He represents Man stretched to the limit of his capacity. Like Apollo he has a chariot, but it stays firmly on the earth, over-running it victoriously.

He is bright as day, hard, straight and sharp as a sword. Optimistic, persistent and brutal, he disregards the future and may spoil it. Grim in decision, sanguine in battle, he is the leader. He is the god of Sword and Action.

Bellona is his sister, driving her chariot while brandishing a whip. She is a busybody. Brother and sister both aim for victory. She is the heroine who leads an army or defends a citadel, an Amazon, an explorer, the helmswoman, the minister at the head of her country's affairs. In a less exalted sphere she is the housewife who pays twenty social calls a day, makes a home for her parents, sorts out her children, and supports her husband in his career. She is Action Woman.

If Saturn and Bacchus seek the Eternal Moment in time; if Jupiter and Apollo pursue Unity and Beauty in space; then Mars aims to break all records and win all contests, whether in war, business, or love. Consider the conquest of peoples, as by Caesar and Napoleon; the subjugation of rebellions, by the Duke of Alba and by Richelieu; and the battles won by such men as Gaston de Foix, the Prince of Condé, and Marshal Foch.

DOMINANT CHARACTERISTICS

Tall stature.
Aggressive demeanour.
Jerky, mechanical gait.
Impulsive, irascible, uncontrolled, violent, angry.

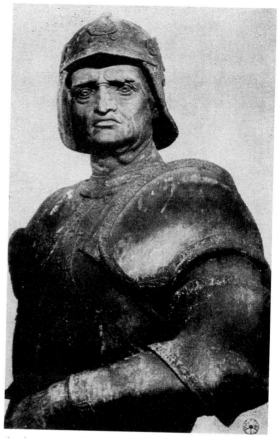

Andrea Verrochio, *Condottiere Colleoni*, (Venice, coll. Anderson-Giraudon)

Description

Very tall (1.80m to 1.95m). Warlike, aggressive stance, with chest thrown out and back strongly braced. Jerky, mechanical gait, with frequent quick gestures, 'date-shaped' face.

The forehead recedes, is often low and always narrow. The occiput is well-developed and projects backwards, giving a dolichocephalic skull.

The nose is curved and very long, like an eagle's beak. The mouth is like a bow, with thin tight lips, but the lower lip is the thicker of the two. The chin curves upwards to meet the nose. The ears are small, and stick out. The hair is reddish. Thick coarse eyebrows tend to meet one another. Greenish eyes, with bloodshot conjunctivae. Brick-red complexion. Short-waisted, with bulging torso. Solid muscular arms. Large strong hands. Long, lean, muscular legs. Large taut feet.

MORPHOLOGY

Static

The Marsian is a large man, the tallest of all the types described. He also gives the greatest impression of strength, because of his muscular development and lively, self-confident, often aggressive attitude. This is an essential characteristic; even in repose the Marsian assumes authority and always seeks to dominate his surroundings.

Consider his face. It is long, narrow and 'date-shaped'. The skull is dolicocephalic, almost pointed at the vertex. The occiput juts out, and in contrast, the forehead recedes. Everything suggests that the cerebration of this individual takes place below the level of consciousness. Indeed, Mars is an instinctive being whose violent reactions are an immediate response to impressions which the subject does not pause to consider. His forehead is often low, always narrow, and prematurely lacking hair; his temples are large, prominent, and rich in blood-vessels which swell and throb at the slightest anger.

His hair is thick and harsh, sometimes curly or fuzzy, and of an auburn or carroty hue. Your redhead is usually a Marsian.

The eyebrows are curved, thick, and very close to the eyes. They easily set in a frown, and are sometimes raised and lowered alternately.

His eyes are wide open, sparkling, lively, of a yellow or tawny colour that turns green in the heat of anger. The conjunctivae are frequently bloodshot. When a Marsian talks to you he fixes you with an unblinking gaze. His glance is firm, bold, hard, fearfully fascinating.

His nose is characteristically aquiline. Prominent at the root, it curves downwards like an eagle's beak. The firm angular tip terminates in a point, below which quiver the wide, dilated nostrils.

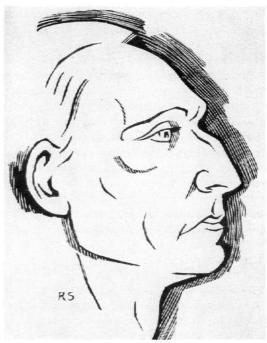

His large, well-formed, disdainful mouth is shaped like a bow, tightly closed by deeply-coloured, passionate thin lips. The lower lip, thicker and redder than the upper, displays a feral pout which gives an impression of ill-humour, even in repose.

His square chin juts forward like a boot. Hooked nose and jutting chin, these are hallmarks of the Marsian. When he gets old and loses his teeth, his nose and chin come even nearer to one another. To quote an old saying, 'The nose makes merry with the chin'. Such was the profile of the wicked fairy Carabosse.

His ears are small and well-shaped and stick out from his head. They are firm, and brick-red or brown in colour.

His cheekbones are prominent, his cheeks muscular, his complexion brick-red. Rust-coloured patches are scattered here and there on his face, especially on the nose. His neck is short, strong, well-muscled and heavily veined.

His shoulders are large, muscular, square, and thrown back, and the upper part of his body often carries branny patches. Marsian women have firm round breasts, but when the arms are extended the breasts look more like well-developed pectoral muscles.

His loins are always strongly braced, the hips hard and bony. His limbs are muscular, large-boned and strong. His arms terminate in hard hands with strong fingers and prominent muscles. The first phalanx of the thumb, which represents the will, is better developed than the second. The nails are short, the fingers spatulate. The mount of Mars is high, and the plain of Mars is crossed by lines pointing in all directions.

By comparison with his short torso, his legs are long, lean, hard and muscular, with the quick action of a trooper or hiker. The feet are large and taut.

Kinetic

The Marsian stance is characteristic – threatening head held high, shoulders braced back, chest thrown forwards. He walks at a brisk, purposeful pace, with an insolent, provocative bearing. Slow in greeting, the handshake is hard and energetic. The Marsian woman is candid but ungainly. It is embarrassing to

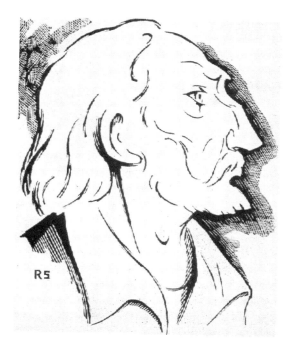

RS

accompany her in the street, because she walks fast and jostles anyone who gets in her way.

A Marsian always walks rapidly. His gestures are sudden and often unexpected. Every movement stems from a sensation he has not had time to analyse. Rapid and abrupt, they astonish by their brutality, even when this arises out of a desire to help, and not as the result of irritation or contradiction. Thus a friend may snatch from you an object you are cleaning, or a piece of work upon which you are engaged, with the sole desire of helping you.

The Marsian has a particularly unpleasant voice – shrill, harsh, vibrating, nasal, resounding and loud. His speech is jerky, his laugh unbearably noisy. Marsians talk very loudly when imparting their opinions. They wish to dominate others and are irritated by contradiction.

Such is the Marsian man in action. The female Marsian lacks gracefulness, and her gestures might be those of a man. She walks quickly, swinging her shoulders. The arrogance of her gait protects her from being followed or accosted. The least observant of men would not risk approaching her for fear of a rebuff.

FUNCTIONS OF THE TYPE

Two things must be noted about the Marsian – his mental and intellectual characteristics, and his character.

Mind

Impulse is the motive force of the Marsian, in whom instinct is the predominant quality. Physiologically irritable, he reacts immediately to the slightest stimulus, the smallest setback, often with a crisis of great violence.

The Marsian mentality is that of a soldier or militant. His attitude is 'aggressive', 'combative', 'systematically contradictory' or 'illogical'. His intelligence is a manifestation of instinct, and is more likely to have been developed in battle than by reflective study. Marsians are very impressionable, irritable people, and their reaction to any stimulus is instantaneous, and violent if anger has been provoked. If on the other hand the stimulus was a pleasant one, the reaction is marked by an explosion of joy which can be heard for miles.

They are impetuous people, incapable of dissimulation unless they have been taught to use it as a strategy. In this case they are crafty and lie low until overcome by anger, when they forget the role they forced themselves to play, and give vent to insults and blind force.

Marsians have a good memory, which often serves to replace intelligence and allows them the reputation of brilliance. Moreover, it is difficult to have a serious discussion with a Marsian, because from the start he becomes angry, talks loudly, rapidly and continuously, often repeating the same words over and over again. He almost stutters in his haste to express his opinion which, more often than not, has been reached neither by thought nor by wisdom, but is purely the expression of an instinct.

Marsians will quarrel over anything, often for no cause other than an interior, unrecognised malaise. If one attempts to hold their attention, in order to argue or reason with them, there is no hope of having the last word. But if you oppose their fury with coldness, indifference or sang-froid, they are at first choked with surprise and indignation, unable to articulate a word. Astounded and discountenanced, they soon collapse. They may go on raging inwardly, but cannot continue to rant and gesticulate.

They need opposition in order to stimulate their instinctive force. An intellectual person with Marsian traits never works so well as when he has an opponent whom he must win over. Then he will prepare a plan of action and marshal his arguments; progressively, ideas that were previously confused and unrelated will become clear in his mind.

In general, Marsians philosophise with fisticuffs, and use striking (in the literal sense of the word) arguments to demonstrate the force of their reason. They are untroubled by scruples and admit but one virtue – Honour – pressed home at the sword's point. Energetic, audacious

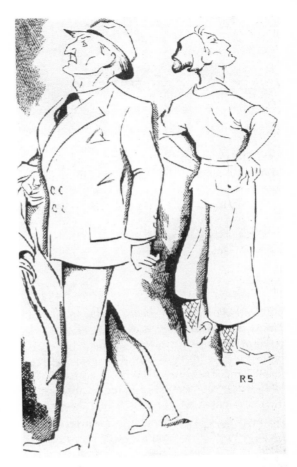

and reckless, they have a steadfast will, indomitable courage and daring, and a contempt for death which enables them to face great danger without fear. They are ready to die for the glory gained by some spectacularly dangerous action, and to risk their own lives unhesitatingly in order to save others.

They can be big-hearted, worthy, magnanimous. They will not hit an enemy when he is down. If he has fallen and is at their mercy, they may grant him his life, but without forgiving him. They have the ideals and virtues of warriors. They are impatient of regulations, but know, none the less, how to submit to military discipline, and severely repress any infraction of it by their subordinates. They exercise power with authority but also with justice. In the

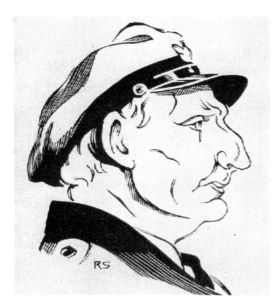

very loudly in order to impose his own opinions, seeks to suppress those of others, and is angry when gainsaid. Vain and proud, he is inclined to glorify his own deeds and belittle those of others.

Given to anger, his rage is sudden, terrible and devastating. During these outbursts he may reach the point of striking the person he is talking to, or if any vestige of self-control remains to him, he will attack surrounding objects or hurl a vase to the ground, reducing it to fragments. Marsian rages do not last for long but their violence is impressive, and their subject often inspires real terror in those around. Actually, these explosions are necessary to the Marsian, helping him to maintain his always unstable equilibrium; it could be said that his nervous system is nourished by anger. These outbursts are easily handled – either give the subject a good hiding, meet force with force, or do not respond at all, remain impassive, let him shout, rant and smash without opposition. Eventually he will calm down, because he is soon exhausted, and the episode will often end in a bilious attack. The rages of the Marsian often mask his weakness, and in the long run produce more noise than damage. It can also be laughable. Mars becomes Punch and his female counterpart the fairy Carabosse, and in old age their noses and chins come together like nutcrackers.

What you must understand about the behaviour of the Marsian is his lack of control, which shows in every aspect of his life. Impatient and rough, he does not look after his clothes but stains and tears them. His first, and noble, instinct is to champion the cause of the weak. Thus he will not allow a child to be beaten, unless he is angry with it, in which case he will lash out blindly at it himself. He likes to take sides in disputes and arguments, and in his generosity will support the weaker side. Mars is to be seen in Don Quixote, as well as in those individuals who express themselves entirely through action.

The Marsian loves the army and military parades. Uniforms fascinate him, war is his

application of law they are merciless, meting out punishment with excessive rigour. Hard to the point of inhumanity, they are unacquainted with pity, but have the gift of inspiring respect and fear by their presence.

They are naturally incredulous, although if they are believers their religious enthusiasm becomes a sort of fanaticism which enables them to brave the torments of death to profess their faith. Their religion, like their other opinions, is demonstrated by energy and action. Their convictions have the strength of instinct and are always accompanied by intolerance. When they pray they bow their heads with reluctance, rarely kneel, and usually just incline their bodies slightly before the Divine Majesty.

Improvident and without forethought, they are very prodigal. Possessions have no meaning for them; only action, above all warlike action, brings them the joys they desire. They like to be noticed, and allowing for the fact that their social class will determine their choice of language, are arrogant and always insolent.

Character

The Marsian is passionate in all he does, for good or ill. He is brutally candid. Violent and petulant, crushing and sharp in speech, he talks

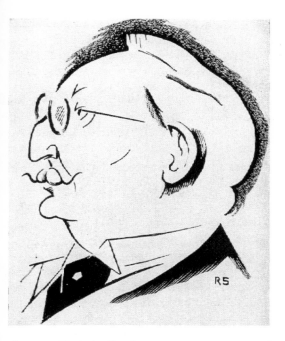

Displays of strength and physical prowess arouse their enthusiasm.

Marsians are also ardent gamblers but do not like losing, and disputes often arise for no other reason than the bad faith of the gambler.

THE MARSIAN WOMAN

In youth the female Marsian is sometimes pretty, but soon begins to develop masculine traits. Her temperament is obvious even in adolescence – she cannot bear to be corrected by her parents and lacks respect for them, and nothing can quell her anger once it is aroused. She has no self-control and the least dissent or contradiction will inflame her to fury. She will fight tooth and nail, but her bark is worse than her bite, for whilst she may be verbally rude and insulting, physical violence quickly gives way to a state of collapse. She cries loudly, laughs boisterously, sobs with rage and complains about trifles. She lacks the patience even to listen to her child repeat its lessons. Her love is formidable, and is carried out like a military operation. She literally captures the man she has chosen, usually a gentle Venusian who cannot resist her. Her jealousy is terrifying; she

element. He is inclined to exaggerate reports of bad news, and despite himself, derives a secret satisfaction at the thought or sight of catastrophes and disasters. In troubled times, when law and order are no longer respected, the pitiless character of the Marsian manifests itself as a desire to kill.

On the other hand, invasion shows him at his best. A true patriot, he loves his native land and will defend it at all costs. Deeds of astounding bravery were done by Marsian members of the French Resistance.

A Marsian is much inclined to the pleasures of love. He is bold with women, but inconstant. His favourite is the Venusian, whose voluptuous langour enchants him. The myth tells all: Mars cuckolds Vulcan with Venus. Venus loves Mars the chivalrous hero, not the mindless bravo who fights whatever enemy presents himself. Note here that Marsians themselves do not forgive a breach of conjugal faith. Othello was a Marsian.

Big eaters and drinkers, they will do justice to a meal of any size. Works of art are lost on them; but noisy spectacular musicals, prize-fights, racing, gymnastic displays, cockfighting or bullfighting will prove an irresistible draw.

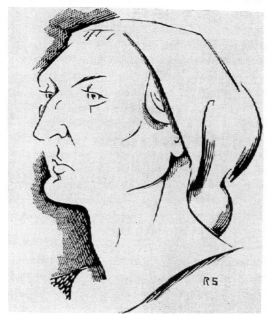

can kill in a fit of rage. However unreasonably, she exacts the outward signs of submission from her husband or lover and takes pleasure in humiliating him. Even if she marries a fellow Marsian she will dominate him, and ridicule him in public.

The Marsian woman knows no fear. Her first instinct is to defend the weak, and in a catastrophe or disaster she will act with courage and devotion. Faithful in misfortune, generous in prosperity, she will lend on request, without security; she brings presents for her friends each time she returns from a journey. The Marsian woman has a large soul and a strong sense of her own dignity. She is boastful and readily despises those around her. She must always be right, and her method of discussion is to raise, first her voice and then her hand, and she may even smash something. She does not lie – in her aggressiveness she prefers to snub people, talk straight and hammer home the point. A threat hovers about her lips, ready for the slightest contradiction.

Her enemies are numerous and tenacious, so often and so unjustly does she wound even those she loves. The devotion she shows in moments of danger cannot compensate for her despotic and brutal moods. Mother-love is a heroic quality in the Marsian woman, and she would endure privation in order to give her children a good upbringing.

She dresses in bright colours, especially shades of red. Blue bores her. Her hats are loaded with plumes and cockades, and one of her favourite luxuries is fur, on others as well as on herself. Despotic and quick-tempered, the Marsian woman lacks charm. She is a dauntless virago, sometimes seductive, but never easy to live with, whimsical but aggressive towards anyone who cannot curb her. Like her Saturnian sister she is better avoided, unless by an explorer or adventurer who could involve her in a life so full of hard work and danger as to make good use of her energy. Then she would become a trusted companion, faithful unto death. In ordinary life she represents nothing but trouble and strife.

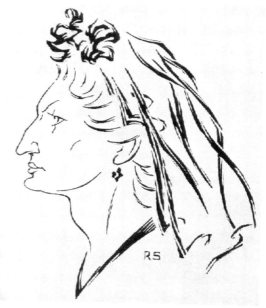

To conclude, Marsians are impulsive, brave, bold, violent, authoritarian and proud. Their warlike aptitudes are incontestable. Action, and above all combat, is their purpose, whether as soldier, politician or priest. Their careers are usually not long, but filled with glory and excitement, and they know how to confront the blows of adversity with a fearless soul. Their deaths may be unexpected and violent, often as a result of their devotion or foolhardiness.

'Mars is clean as daylight, hard, straight and sharp as a sword, tanned by the sun, joyous as the future. Choleric in decision, sanguine in attack, he is the Leader. Hopeful, hard-working and rough, he loves children and noise. His sin is anger. He disregards the future and does violence to it, and sometimes he falls, suddenly cut off by a stroke.'

DISEASES AND REMEDIES OF THE MARSIAN

The characteristics of the Marsian are modified by the constitution of the individual, and can also be changed by the illnesses from which he may suffer. The prototype Mars, as described, gives some idea of temperament and character, but its variations must be studied according to the constitutional type to which the subject belongs. Temperament may be modified by constraint or education, but constitution is unalterable, presenting an indelible pattern of build and behaviour which does not change.

Carbonic Constitution

Stubborn and obstinate, the individual does what he wants to do, listens neither to advice nor comment, even if justified, and goes his own way. If he is intelligent, he applies his will to a purpose, wishing to work and to succeed. Energetic, although hard and unsympathetic, he is never moved by sentiment, uses all his efforts to succeed, and tolerates no opposition.

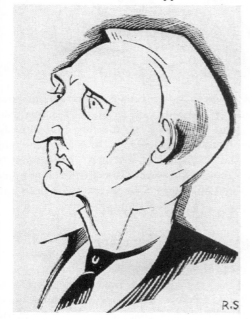

R.S

Phosphoric Constitution

An egotist who fancies himself, knowing that he is superior to those around him, whom he regards with scorn and disgust. He feels so far above them that they cannot comprehend his superiority. Avid for glory, he makes his will known merely by saying, 'I shall do such-and-such', but as he is also unreflecting, he is liable to run into difficulties he had not even suspected of existing, and his idealism, woven from

dreams and lacking common sense, may lead him to smarting failure.

Fluoric Constitution

The need to dominate, which animates every Marsian subject, leads him to act on impulse. Intelligent and very observant, he sees in a flash the faults of his adversary and knows how to exploit them. With irresistible authority he takes over any situation; he is at once in command, for he knows how to gain respect. Unfortunately his overbearing attitude is associated with a certain truculence which renders him insufferable to thoughtful people. He wants to succeed, and he must succeed quickly, for despite his appetite for admiration he also tires easily. But he is fond of money, and needs it urgently to finance his desire for power and outward show, and a lack of forethought often leads him to commit actions which are definitely compromising.

TRANSMUTATIONS OF THE MARSIAN

Among those authors who have described human Types minutely in astral or planetary terms, there has been established a subtle distinction between 'Auspicious' and 'Inauspicious' types. We consider that no such distinction should be made, and that it is artificial and may be misleading. The inauspicious aspect of Mars arises through exaggeration of his natural qualities. Accentuated tendencies become vile faults; excessive passion is seen as vice, and violent behaviour always as murderous. In fact, the inauspicious aspect of Mars arises when we see him at his worst – this relates not only to moral turpitude but also to the diseases which may affect him.

Modifications of the Type

In the 'bad Marsian' or the 'inauspicious' aspect of Mars, the facial characters are seen to advantage. The forehead has scarcely developed, so low and receding it is; the deep eyes, hidden behind thick eyebrows, are green and bloodshot. The mouth, with corners turned well down, is set in an almost lipless grin. He has red hair. His voice is loud and harsh. The appearance of this individual is sinister and terrifying. He walks with big strides, fists clenched, shoulders swinging, casting to left and right of him a furious, insolent and provocative glare, seeking whom he may devour. Threats and abuse pour ceaselessly from his mouth. You will meet with such a character among the dregs of society. Seekers after quarrels, instigators of fights, they are redoubtable because of both their strength and their ferocity. They can be seen at times of social unrest, collecting at street corners, promulgating mob law which knows but one rule – violence.

Obscene and lustful, they wallow in debauchery and take pleasure in orgies. They despise and insult all that is above their understanding, and confident in their own boldness, in their brutal strength and the terror which they inspire, laugh scornfully at human justice. Nonetheless, many of them have lost their heads on the scaffold in punishment for their crimes.

At a higher social level the tendency is the same, although it may be masked by early education. At his deepest level the Marsian is always a man of blood, though he is not inevitably fated to become an assassin. Butchers, lumberjacks and surgeons often have a lot of Mars in their make-up.

The 'bad' or 'inauspicious' Marsian woman, when born to high life, enjoys hunting, especially deer, wild boar, and more dangerous beasts; she loves dogs and horses, but cannot stand cats, which she may even kill. She spends a lot of time in the stables, familiar with the grooms, and will sometimes be obscene, cursing and swearing in a raucous voice, without a thought for her reputation.

Lacking self-control, she shuns society, or descends from her social class to live a coarse and independent life with deplorable connections. Due to her stubborn wish to dominate she loses discrimination, and accepts crazy tributes of drink, food and ribaldry. She will risk her life for a challenge, even from strangers.

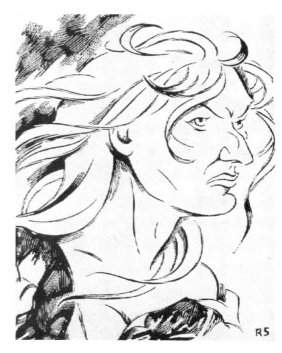

She rejoices in the feelings aroused by her free and easy ways as well as by her tyranny. She destroys everything she touches, both literally and figuratively speaking. Born a woman, she can be tougher than any man. Not content to defy morality in private, she affronts it in broad daylight and threatens society with her misdeeds.

MORBID PREDISPOSITIONS

Psychological Disorders

Just as an alcoholic can suffer from crises of delirium tremens, the Marsian can throw fits of rage such that he loses all control of himself, and little by little, losing his good qualities, turns into a sombre brute beyond hope of redemption. Inauspicious aspect? No. Sickness? Yes. It must be emphatically stated that the bad Marsian is still a Marsian, but an exaggerated version, intoxicated by environmental or chemical poisons, who has lost his good qualities, retaining only those vices whose horrifying qualities must not be neglected, since they are destructive and lead to crime.

Physical Disorders

Physically the Marsian is a 'muscle man' who needs to use his strength and also to restore it. He eats a lot, especially large quantities of meat, at every meal. The output of physical energy which he enjoys – and needs – to use, means that he must replace it with abundant nourishment, mainly of highly seasoned food. He drinks a lot – not water, which he does not care for – but strong alcoholic drinks, full-bodied wines, aperitifs, brandy and liqueurs. After a good meal he feels better, in balance as it were, but this peaceful state of affairs does not last long, for he livens up at the least argument and loses his temper at the slightest contradiction.

The Marsian easily becomes congested; he is also bilious, and his liver suffers from the assaults which its owner does not spare it, since he is hard put to digest and eliminate all the food and drink he consumes.

The heart and the liver are the Marsian's two weak spots. Look around you and note the 'bilious attacks' which follow rage – rather than emotional shocks, grief or worry – and you will almost always find that the patient presents the

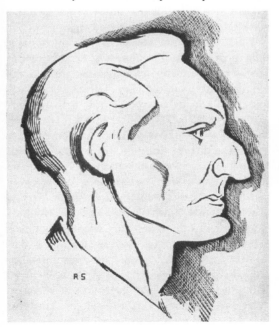

qualities of a Marsian. Sudden congestions, ruptured blood vessels, embolisms, are his likely fate. Not infrequently he also becomes an alcoholic.

TREATMENT

Two deep-acting remedies are commonly indicated in the Marsian subject: Sulphur and Lycopodium.

Sulphur

Sulphur is the first remedy that comes to mind for a sanguine, congested individual who eats and drinks to excess, and who is accustomed to denying himself nothing and doing everything he wants without restriction. Failure to stick to his diet is the rule, auto-intoxication the result. A Marsian will indeed often show the indications for Sulphur – need for fresh air, horror of heat, exacerbation of hunger pains, irritating eruptions alternating with haemorrhoids whose discharge brings momentary relief. The centrifugal action of Sulphur encourages the elimination of toxins that is so necessary to ensure, at least temporarily, the organic equilibrium of the subject.

Excessive eating and drinking by the Marsian

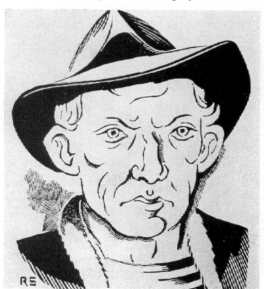

is at the origin of the circulatory troubles that lead him to present with arterial hypertension and the resulting vascular accidents for which Sulphur is often indicated. But in truth, Sulphur can as easily be the remedy for other prototypes who present with signs of auto-intoxication. Often in the course of a chronic disease the patient will report a number of symptoms whose repertorisation appears to be very different, and we are led to prescribe Sulphur which, according to Nash, 'will clarify the case'.

Lycopodium

The basic constitutional remedy of Mars is Lycopodium. Do not forget that the Marsian is always 'liverish'. This is inevitable, not only because of his habitual overeating but also because of the stress he undergoes as a result of his numerous altercations. Added to this will be his propensity to alcoholism.

We must abandon the theoretical notion which seemed to guide us earlier when we considered the indications for Sulphur, the major remedy for auto-intoxication. There is nothing against giving Sulphur, but the idea of Lycopodium may seem bizarre. Lycopodium is that moss with long fronds which, in late autumn, sheds a scentless powder with many uses. A brief examination of some of the characteristics of this remedy will serve to

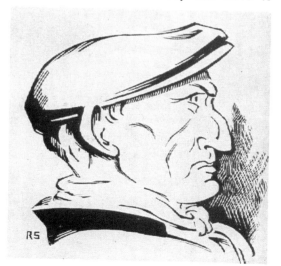

justify its use in the Marsian.

The Lycopodium subject is sensitive and irritable. Sensitivity – he is easily vexed. A word, a gesture, even a look is enough to annoy him. This individual is difficult to handle – you never know which end to start with, since the slightest opposition is likely to bring on a bilious attack which presents not merely with biliary colic but with more or less severe hepatic pain. This is followed by objective signs – yellow face, pale stools, dark urine. The patient really suffers before he recovers, until another crisis provokes a return of the same trouble. Such is the cause of many 'gallbladder attacks'. Surgery can do nothing (except remove gallstones) to prevent a recurrence of this situation, due to a spasmodic condition to which the Marsian is singularly predisposed.

Irritability – extremely irritable, the Lycopodium subject often drives himself into sudden outbursts of anger, exploding with rage. He loses all self-control, using coarse language and violent gestures. If circumstances force him to restrain himself, he at once becomes ill. His liver reacts and soon afterwards he develops a painful hepatic crisis.

His habitual irritability shows in his face, his gait, his movements, words and writing.

The Lycopodium subject looks much older than he really is. Prematurely deep wrinkles furrow his habitually severe countenance, giving him the look of an old man. This is particularly remarkable in babies. His gait is active, quick and anxious, lacking in elasticity. He often clicks his heels whilst walking. Movements are exaggerated and incoherent, words violent. Incapable of expressing himself gently, he stresses every word, sometimes even every syllable; he talks vehemently, often carried away by what he is saying, and his listeners could believe him to be angry when in fact he is only seeking to make himself clear. It is certainly true that he cannot stand argument or opposition, which are likely to provoke from him a lively response, or even a fit of anger.

He writes as he speaks, using violent language that is seldom accurate, often vulgar and coarse,

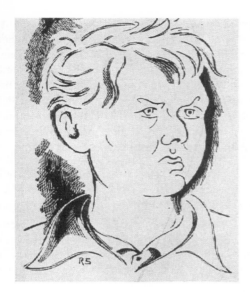

underlining with an authoritarian flourish those words which most strongly express his meaning. His writing usually slopes backwards.

This nervous irritability – surely of toxic origin – continues during sleep. The patient starts in his sleep, often dreams of accidents, and generally wakes in a bad humour so that he begins the day by grumbling. It is the same throughout life: the baby screams all day and is only quiet at night; the adult shouts at people even when they are being friendly. Women have increased tension before periods, but the irritability becomes most obvious and unbearable in old people who have 'authoritarian crises', coupled with cerebral weakness and loss of memory. They cannot find words with which to express themselves, and when writing they forget letters, and sometimes a whole word.

From this collection of characteristic symptoms, extracted from the homoeopathic materia medica, we derive a speaking likeness of the usual behaviour of the Marsian. No remedy could fit our subject better, and we are thus made aware of the immense relevance of homoeopathy, the only discipline which takes account of temperament: truly, a human medicine.

The Marsian is often if not always a liverish subject. Consider the child: from time to time he is odious to his parents, disagreeable with his companion, then suddenly runs a temperature and vomits. The characteristic smell of his breath denotes an attack of acidosis whose periodicity accompanies the functional changes in his liver. An adult frequently complains of right hypochondrial discomfort with heaviness and swelling; he cannot lie on his right side, his liver is sensitive and tender. Here are the characteristic symptoms of Lycopodium. The similarity is closer when objective signs associated with the remedy make their appearance: skin scattered with liver-spots, a yellowish tint in the face with typical darker patches in the temporal regions, a reduction of urinary nitrogen. However, it would be a great mistake to adopt the oversimplified formula that Mars = Lycopodium. Sulphur and Lycopodium may be the deep-acting remedies that suit the Marsian, but there are other, auxiliary remedies which should not be neglected.

Consider the typical behaviour of the Marsian subject: all his actions are violent and show a total lack of self-control. Anger is for him not just a bad mistress; it dominates his life by creating disturbances in the play of his functions, with varying results. This situation is well-known to homoeopaths, who are able to determine which of the patient's complaints can be attributed to his temperament, and find in the materia medica those remedies that are appropriate for him.

Without a doubt the remedies for anger and its bad effects will be those most often prescribed for the Marsian. The morbid conditions which we have to treat are not always due to an external cause, whether microbial or atmospheric. The patient too often carries within himself the reason for the complaints that he submits to us for diagnosis.

Nux Vomica
Certainly Nux Vomica will frequently be used in conjunction with Sulphur or Lycopodium, either to improve functional digestive disorders or to reduce the hypersensitivity of a patient

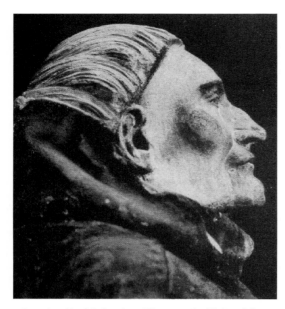

Antoine Le Moiturier, *Thomas de Plaine* (circa 1745), detail (Masterpieces of the Louvre, gothic heads, Editions Calavas)

who has been over-indulging in stimulants such as coffee, tea, wine, spirits and aperitifs. Nux Vomica cannot bear the slightest sound, bright lights or strong smells. He cannot tolerate contradiction or opposition. A violent man, he 'blows up' easily, shouting insults and losing control of himself. A nap, however short, will bring instant improvement.

Anacardium

The Anacardium subject, with unbalanced will subject to contradictory impulses, and a suspicious, nasty character, flies into violent tempers. He cannot contain himself, and whatever his social status, uses bad language, cursing, swearing, blasphemy and obscene words. His attitude improves whilst he is eating a meal.

Chamomilla

Chamomilla is often indicated in the infant Mars. Even as a baby he shows a strong will, wants to be given in to, and if denied, flies into a temper that results in convulsions. When older he is capricious and self-willed, always discon-

tented, never satisfied. He desires something, and when it is given to him, throws it away and demands something else. Restless, suspicious, grumbling and in bad humour, he cannot bear to be looked at, spoken to or approached, but shouts and jumps up and down with rage. It is valuable to note that this child, who cannot keep still and is altogether impossible, becomes quiet as soon as he is picked up and carried, or pushed around in a pram.

Colocynthis

Colocynth is particularly relevant for the individual who suddenly experiences very violent, cramping, intermittent pain after a fit of anger. This pain is usually peri-umbilical, and is relieved by hard pressure which forces the patient to bend forward. You might be called out in an emergency to find a patient lying as stiff as a gun-dog in his bed, or doubled up over the back of a chair in order to try to relieve the painful cramps from which he is suffering. Before diagnosing appendicitis or renal colic, question the relatives, and you may learn that the patient had a violent altercation with his boss or one of his employees, and that it was after returning home that the pain started.

Gelsemium

Gelsemium is another remedy that suits the Marsian when, after a setback, often of emotional origin, a state of violent irritation supervenes, with fits of anger or indignation. The face is red and congested and the patient complains of a curious sensation – 'as if the heart would stop beating unless he keeps moving'. It seems as if movement is needed to keep the organism alive. Later the patient has an attack of trembling or urgent diarrhoea, and finally there may be a state of depression with insomnia lasting for several hours or even days.

Aurum Metallicum

The Aurum patient is congested and sanguine, but he is also a hypersensitive person who sees the dark side of everything and is easily annoyed. Always preoccupied, never content,

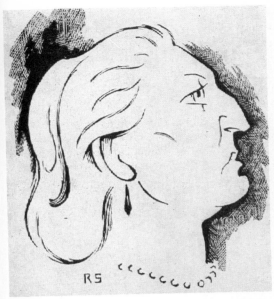

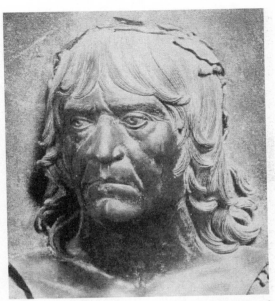

Sperandi Miglioli, *Mantegna* (Mantua, Church of Saint Andrew, photo Alinari-Giraudon)

he is very irritable. He cannot bear the slightest contradiction, which provokes mad rages – veritable explosions, which upset all those around him – and which he later regrets. Aurum is an excellent remedy for the hypertensive Marsian, especially when he shows signs of aortitis, so frequent in the bearers of hereditary specific (syphilitic) disease (Fluorics).

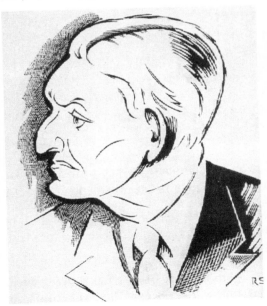

Staphysagria

For the sake of completeness we should include Staphysagria, the remedy for suppressed anger, although in fact it is not often prescribed for the Marsian, who usually expresses his feelings violently. More often we need to have recourse to one of the remedies previously cited: Nux Vomica, Anacardium, Chamomilla, Colocynth, Gelsemium or Aurum, whose characteristics are so often discerned in the habitual behaviour of the Marsian complex.

Spiritus Quercus Glandium

Finally, do not forget that Mars is often an alcoholic who needs Spiritus Quercus Glandium, whose action is specific in alcoholic intoxication.

Life Style

The impulsive character of Mars makes it difficult for him to lead a regular life. He does what comes to mind, and though he can accept a rigorous military discipline, finds it almost impossible to discipline himself in ordinary civilian life. In view of his habitual violence it is

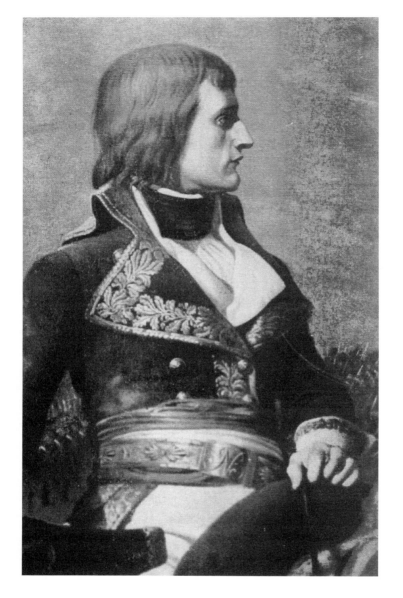

Philippoteaux, *Bonaparte at the Battle of Rivoli*, detail (Versailles Museum, photo Bulloz)

necessary to 'break him in', and you will not obtain peace except by imposing vigorous physical exercise, which will help to restore the balance.

Diet must not be neglected. Abstention from meat on certain days and reduction or even total suppression of alcoholic drinks will make things easier, but if the conditions are too strict the subject will rebel.

The Marsian must be well provisioned. He requires substantial and stimulating meals on account of his muscular build and expenditure of energy. He has a further need – that of becoming angry, which for him is a means of feeding his nervous system.

The Marsian is aggressive, impulsive, violent and rough. An open-air life with plenty of exercise is necessary to maintain his equilibrium, and to counter, by the compensatory effect of daily muscular fatigue, his natural irritability and bad temper. To keep a Marsian indoors is to bring the devil into the house. A child will break the furniture, a man will batter his wife, and the wife will murder her husband. Fortunately, pure Mars types are rarely met with in present-day society. They make their appearance in times of trouble, during wars and catastrophes. The outstanding quality of Mars is action inspired by impulse, his greatest fault is anger inflamed by pride. He rarely pauses to reflect, and is always active. For him, 'Might is Right'.

MARS: THE REMEDIES

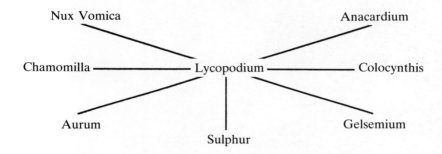

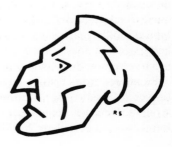

5

Saturn

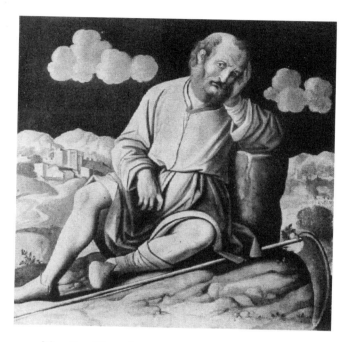

Mocetto, *Time*, fragment (collection Jacquemart-André, photo Bulloz)

Artists wishing to depict the idea of Time and the sedentary life use as their model a tall, thin, bent and sad old person, with a long bony face, strongly accentuated features, dark flat lustreless hair, a narrow forehead, a long straight nose which dives vertically towards the mouth, lined cheeks and dull, dreary eyes. Saturn, the typical intellectual, spreads his wings in boundless space and does not touch Earth until his life is harvested by the scythe of Time.

Examples from history include Henry II of France, Cosimo de Medici, Catherine of Aragon, Heinrich Heine, Leopold, King of the Belgians, and President Woodrow Wilson.

DOMINANT CHARACTERISTICS

Tall stature.
Weary drooping posture, prematurely aged.
Slow and awkward gait.
Taciturn, gloomy, egoistic, always a pessimist.

DESCRIPTION

Tall (height 1.80–1.90m in men; 1.70–1.80m in women). Sad, old, weary appearance. Long, thin and bent. Slow, flat-footed gait.

Seated, he rests his elbow on his knee and his chin in his hand. The face is the shape of an almond. High forehead, domed and narrow.

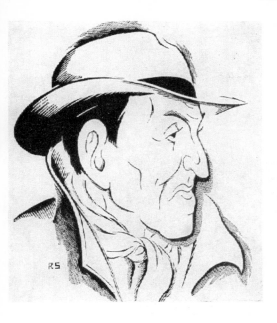

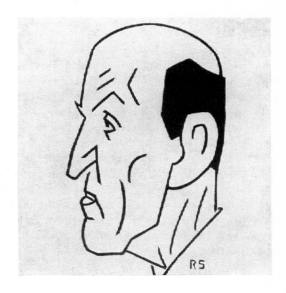

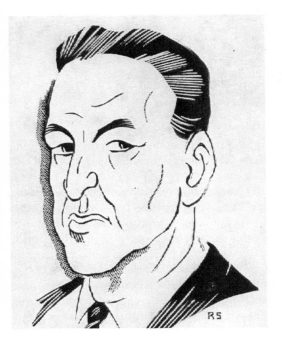

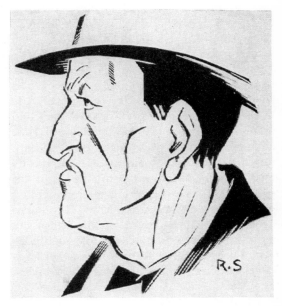

Flat occiput. Dolicocephalic. Long narrow nose which almost touches the upper lip. Large wide mouth, turned down at the corners. The lower lip often projects in front of the upper lip.

Square chin, like a horse's jaw. Big smooth ears, flattened against the skull. Dark, lustreless straight hair. Sallow complexion. Narrow bony chest, indrawn belly. Long hands and feet.

MORPHOLOGY

Static

The Saturnian is always tall and thin, with big bones, rigid, powerful, thickened joints and palpable dilated veins. His skin is generally yellowish-brown, firm, dry, cold and hairy.

At first sight the observer is struck by a characteristic lack of proportion, made more obvious by the typical thinness of the Saturnian. He is tall, with big bones, but his chest is narrow and indrawn. The women have flat breasts. The shoulders are narrow and curved, the arms and legs are long, the hips bony, massive and projecting. The total effect is of inharmonious disproportion.

Consider first the face: it is shaped like an almond, with the point at the top, and a square chin. The skull is vaulted with a domed vertex, and usually dolicocephalic. The face in profile is almost rectangular. The occiput is flat, the temples smooth and regressive, the high, narrow, bulging forehead is almost square, crossed by horizontal lines, with a V between the eyebrows that is more marked when the subject is lost in thought.

The hair is very dark, straight, greasy, often damp, and with clubbed ends. Its growth is sparse in places. Baldness is frequent and early in the Saturnian. The eyebrows are dark and quite a distance away from the eyes. They almost meet at the root of the nose, and are raised like circumflex accents. The eyebrows tend to project forwards, forming a sort of eyeshade.

The eyelids are thick and heavy. The upper eyelid is high and curved, so that when the eyebrow is raised the forehead folds into horizontal lines (mask of Saturn). The lower lid is large, thick and puffy, and folds into wrinkles. The eyelashes are dark, coarse and sparse.

The eyes are very dark and deep-set. They are dull and gloomy, devoid of light and brilliance, 'like pools of stagnant water', according to Petrarch. The conjunctivae are yellowish (prune-eyed). The gaze lacks fire and is marked by lassitude and sadness. Usually

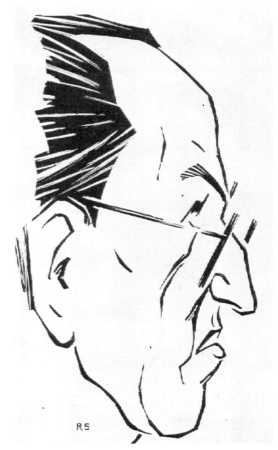

withdrawn and serious, it can become piercing when fixed upon something or in the heat of a discussion.

The nose is large, bony, projecting, very long, thin at the tip, and falls away steeply towards the mouth, almost touching the upper lip. The nostrils are ample and so thick that they appear to be closed, the tip of the nose forming the apex of a triangle. The mouth is large and sullen, with turned-down corners; the naso-labial folds are deeply engraved into the thin, sunken cheeks. The lips are ugly, the lower lip is pendulous and often projects in front of the upper lip.

The chin is square, like a horse's jaw, with a well-defined horizontal line running across it. The beard is very dark, rough, and irregular. The cheek-bones are bony and prominent.

The ears are large and broad, pressed back against the skull, with pendant lower lobes and heavy cartilages.

The neck is long, thin and fleshless, with cord-like muscles and a projecting Adam's Apple.

The chest is narrow and bony. The breasts are virtually non-existent in a Saturnian woman.

The back is thin and bent, with projecting vertebrae, the shoulders high, square and visibly bony, with winged scapulae. The long, poorly-muscled arms end in long thin hands with prominent tendons, leading to bony fingers with projecting joints.

The belly is concave, the thighs flat, bony and thin, the legs slender, wasted and often hairy. The feet are flat and bony and the veins on them stand out; the heels are broad and flat.

Kinetic

The characteristic attitude of the Saturnian reflects his discouragement with life. In the standing position the arms hang down beside the body, the head pokes forward or to one side, the back is bent, and he often leans on a walking-stick as if he lacked the equilibrium to support himself. The Saturnian looks old – older than his years – but is long-lived because he knows how to conserve his strength.

Seated, the Saturnian crosses his legs and rests an elbow on his knee, holding his chin in a hand whose thumb is extended whilst the fingers are folded over the palm. Thus he provides his own natural support, as usual slightly bent forward, an attitude which may denote either weariness or deep thought. When lying down, the Saturnian supports himself on one elbow, either the right or the left, in order to think or to read.

The gait of a Saturnian may be slow, grave, timid or embarrassed, or a combination of these. Often he may be seen advancing with head bent forward and eyes fixed upon the ground, talking to himself, apparently absorbed in deep and sometimes bitter thought. His gestures are either infrequent and clumsy, because his joints lack suppleness, or else thoughtful, slow, meaningful and repeated.

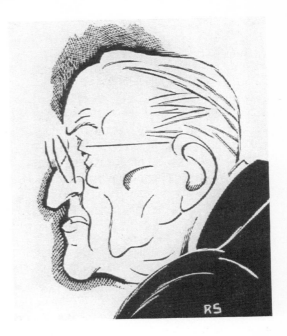

They are neither original nor spontaneous; they may support his arguments, but without ardour or vehemence.

All the movements of a Saturnian are deliberate, unless he is the victim of a nervous disorder that causes a tic. Quite often the Saturnian is demented.

The voice of a Saturnian is low and discordant, fairly resonant and somewhat slurred. The woman has a masculine voice; the man's is deep and almost tragic. A Saturnian always speaks slowly, rarely smiles and never laughs, but may sometimes let slip a sardonic chuckle.

This is the Saturnian, at rest and in motion. He is without elegance or grace, and all the qualities we have noted are uncouth and unattractive. So it is not surprising that the Saturnian woman, too, lacks charm. Whilst the little Saturnian girl may present a certain melancholy sweetness, the adolescent already looks like an old maid. She is never really feminine but belongs to a neuter gender, especially if she is passive; if active, she rapidly becomes masculine. Nonetheless, whilst the Creator may not have endowed the Saturnian woman with charm, he has given her a deep soul and a

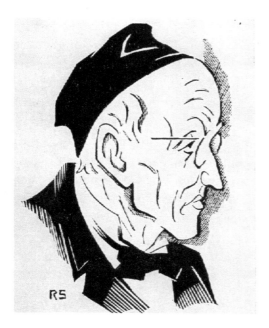

RS

powerful mind. Further study of her attributes will show what an immense store of energy can be contained in her unattractive body.

FUNCTIONS OF THE TYPE

Mind

Logic is the dominant faculty of Saturnians. Intelligent and cultivated, they show a remarkable capacity for pure science, mathematics, philosophy and criticism. They are powerful rationalists, great logicians who revel in controversy. As metaphysicians they erect their concepts into dogmas; as physicists they state axioms which become articles of faith and can then be demonstrated in the abstract by calculation; as biologists or chemists they set themselves to detailed analysis of the elements. In all fields of intellectual activity they aim to demonstrate, by means of reason, principles and facts which their listeners are invited to accept, without discussion of procedures or systems. Methodical classifiers, compulsive planners, Saturnians sometimes create Utopias. Then they destroy the real in favour of the imaginary, whilst others give them credit for being practical because they can manipulate numbers and figures with a skill and boldness which is denied to those less able.

Indefatigable logicians, they deduce all the consequences of a principle which they themselves have erected, a fact they have observed, or an axiom they have accepted. They are intransigeant dogmatists in whatever field they may work. Inclined to hero-worship, to religiosity, to credulity and even to superstition, they carry into the domains of science, sociology, philosophy and literature their need for faith and inquisitorial proselytism.

They are religious by nature, conviction and need; but their souls are constantly tortured by doubts – doubts which may plunge them into bitter despair, even leading them to suicide. Meditative men, profound thinkers, tireless seekers, patient workers, their spirits are never at rest but forever occupied in trying to solve the most serious problems and answer the most difficult and transcendental questions. Above all, they are absorbed by the study of the Divine Essence and the immortality of the soul. These questions, which torment them, also have the greatest fascination for them.

They often contemplate death, even though they fear it greatly. Dying for them is a terrible process, shot through with denial and protest – unless faith, overcoming rebellion, delivers them. In matters of religion they are austere, adopting the starkest forms of asceticism and mortification. When they invoke the Divine Majesty it is with deep fear and respect, genuflecting repeatedly, beating their breasts and prostrating themselves, even to the extent of knocking their heads on the ground.

However, in general, they are characterised by wisdom and prudence. They have a penetrating wit and profound intelligence. At once thoughtful and foresighted, they make excellent counsellors. Their memory is astonishing and durable; the smallest fact is retained and retrieved at the appropriate moment, enabling them, for instance, to recognise immediately a person they have only ever met once.

They manage their affairs with marvellous

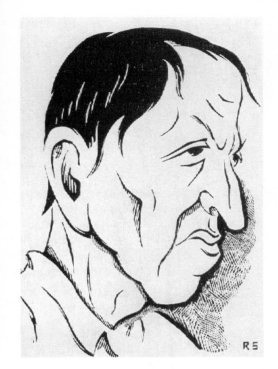

introverts who repress within themselves all sensations and feelings such as grief, guarding in silence the projects they have planned. Consummate politicians and diplomats, by their prudence and perseverance they overcome great difficulties, and know the art of bringing the most sensitive negotiations to a satisfactory conclusion. They never lack the means of extricating themselves from embarrassing situations, and readily seize upon the faults of their adversaries in order to gain advantage. Niggardly in giving promises, they scrupulously observe those which they have made; they are bound by their word.

Once they have made a resolution they are unshakeable in keeping it. The love of independence is theirs in the highest degree, but reason and will enable them to submit to the most rigorous disciplines. They are slaves of the habits which they try to preserve.

Friends of solitude, foes of noise, they are self-sufficient and live alone, shunning the activity of a world they despise. Taciturn or deliberately silent, surly and dejected, quick to

ability, being tenacious in their opinions, persevering in their undertakings, stubborn in the execution of their plans. They will not commit themselves without long reflection, having carefully considered the good and bad results which could ensue.

Art for them is always secondary to science. Music must rest upon abstract calculations which rule out unexpected results and have nothing to do with artistic sensibility. Geometrical drawings mean more to them than the observation of nature or the recording of sense-impressions. In literature they apply themselves to philosophical speculation, discussions on the meaning of words, criticism, or the composition of works full of methodical documentation.

Character

Grave and melancholy slaves of duty, Saturnians speak little, as if they were afraid of wasting their thoughts. They weigh their words, sometimes expressing themselves sententiously. They say no more than is needed. They are

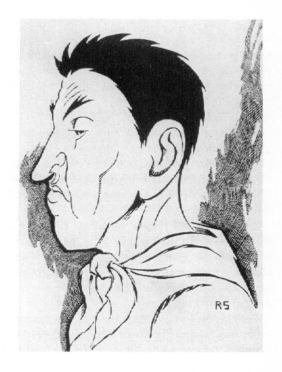

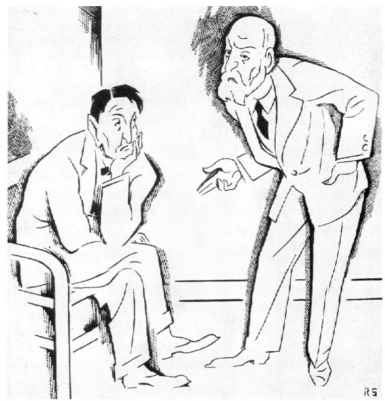

see the worst in everything, to detect ill-will in others, to believe themselves persecuted; distrustful and suspicious, meticulous and obsessive, they emanate misery and by their very presence dispel feelings of joy in those around them.

Egotistical and parsimonious, they hide their gloomy pride and clumsy shyness beneath a cloak of false humility that darkens their surroundings and makes everyone feel ill at ease. Their misanthropy is expressed in sarcasm and despair. Think of Molière's Alceste.

Given their distrust and suspicion, they find it difficult to make friends, but when they do love, it is with deep and enduring devotion. They cherish the memory of offences, forgiving rarely and with effort. They are little stirred by sensual pleasures and make poor lovers.

Ambitious for honours and degrees, rather than for glory and renown, they secretly aspire to wield the highest authority and will spare no

effort to attain it. Among them are famous politicians, with great gifts of managing the affairs of State. Fired with the desire of founding institutions as monuments to their memory, they make sure that these are well constructed to resist the depredations of time.

Saturnians are always industrious; patient and assiduous, they can sustain long, hard work. Amongst them may be found thinkers and philosophers, and the founders of religious orders who through their powerful organisations control society. They also include antiquarians and collectors.

Sadness and pessimism are the two principal qualities of the Saturnian, and these dictate his tastes. He prefers to wear dark, generally black clothes. His rooms feel cold, and the miserliness of the proprietor is evident from the economies he practises. Daylight filters through shutters or thick curtains, leaving the room in almost complete darkness. Lights are turned on only when he has visitors. He is obsessional about the position of familiar objects, sits in the same chair every day and does the same things at the same times, according to an unvarying plan of life. His rooms are sombre with old furniture made from dark or black wood, iron chests, antique tapestries, pictures of lowering landscapes under stormy skies. Saturnians like dark colours, heavy solid furniture, sparsely furnished, lightless, airless rooms. They prefer old (Renaissance) or rustic furniture, but will sometimes break out into the most extraordinary modern creations, depending on whether they are moved by respect for tradition or by love of the bizarre. They are either intransigent conservatives, or revolutionaries determined to make a clean sweep of the past so as to dominate the present and create the conditions for the future.

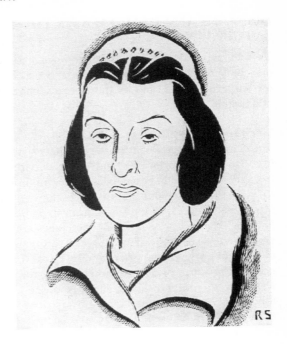

The Saturnian Woman

The female Saturnian is an orderly woman who knows how to run her home, keeps careful accounts, and realises the value of every penny. The Valiant Woman of the Scriptures, who scrutinised her handmaidens, who considered a field and bought it, and who gave everyone their working orders at dawn, must have been a Saturnian. She is a good helpmate, a chaste and faithful wife, but can be peevish, bored and boring. Her devotion is lethal, her affection expressed with jealousy which engulfs its object. She practises exasperating economies. Full of petty precautions, she leaves nothing to chance, keeps her keys in her pockets, burns every scrap of paper which might be compromising, and automatically suspects everyone who greets her.

The Saturnian woman has a masculine intellect and can expect little hope of joy from her body, devoid as it is of feminine grace and beauty. The poor girl seems destined to celibacy from puberty. What rancours must be hidden beneath her narrow flat chest! Nevertheless, if the Saturnienne wants to be loved, and applies her superior intelligence to this purpose, she will achieve it. She possesses in high degree the perseverence which singles out a man, slowly lays siege to him, and finally has her way with him. Her devotion is unequalled; fanatical in love as in religion, her efforts are rewarded with lasting results.

She is born old and dies an octogenarian, like the Saturnian man who is never young, and who drags his obsessions and his sadness through a narrow dreary life which would kill anyone but him. Saturn devours his children so that their father shall live, and the Saturnian woman controls and suppresses all her desires in order to attain unchallenged power. She draws everything and everyone into a chimerical but very real empire.

In conclusion: Saturnians are dominant people, silent, stubborn, sad but persevering. Their habitual attention to detail, their constant complaints, their egoism and their melancholia render them insupportable, but they are still obeyed. Astute Saturn is endowed with prodigious energy. He is the 'Master of Time'. With logic and patience he swallows up everything that claims to live outside his dark despotic realm. He does not bend or break, because he is insensitive to storms and lives within himself.

DISEASES AND REMEDIES OF THE SATURNIAN

The characteristics of the Saturnian, as related, may be modified by the constitution to which the subject belongs, and by the diseases which attack him.

Carbonic Constitution

The Carbonic Saturnian lives an absolutely rigid life. He has his principles and never departs from them, and his habitual logic condemns him to a severe discipline. Hard with himself, intransigeant, accepting no modification to the line of conduct upon which he long ago embarked, he is pitiless with regard to others and never forgives an offence. He thinks of nothing but his work, and knows wonderfully well how to conserve his strength in order to follow his chosen career to an advanced age, even though he is usually pessimistic about the outcome.

Phosphoric Constitution

The dogmatism of a Saturnian, allied to the habitual enthusiasm of a Phosphoric, results in his constructing systems based on artificial axioms created by his own imagination. With faultless logic he will pursue reasoning based on a false premise. He relies on his intuition, which he regards as remarkable and infallible. The exact sciences bore him but he is fascinated by occultism, which allows him to develop without hesitation all his resources of imaginative construction. The disillusionments which follow, and the incomprehension with which he has to struggle, gradually lead him to a dark pessimism which may result in suicide.

Fluoric Constitution

The admirable faculty for assimilation shown by the Fluoric, allied to the passion for detail and logic of the Saturnian, give this subject remarkable qualities which can be turned to good account in the conduct of affairs, diplomatic or financial. But for him the outcome is never satisfactory, especially if he is engaged in financial transactions; he never makes enough

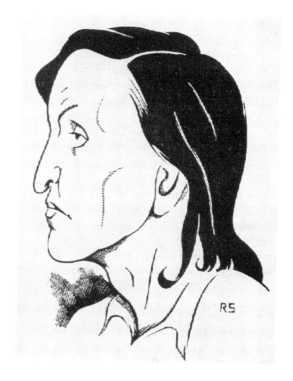

money. His natural stinginess increases with success, and though he may be envied, he is never loved. His life drags on, sad and dreary, despite the wealth he has accumulated.

TRANSMUTATIONS OF THE SATURNIAN

Those authors who have depicted the planetary types felt obliged to describe the propitious and unpropitious aspects of each. In fact the Saturn type has but one description, one morphology, one single human function whose essence we have pointed out. Why describe as unpropitious this Saturn with whose characteristics we are now familiar? Account must be taken of the morphological changes which can be observed in the Saturnian; of the modifications of character, physical alterations and psychological disturbances which can be observed. But all these are simply transmutations of the original type.

Look at a sick person. You will see a healthy

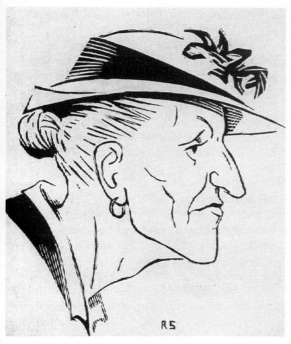

character. It should be easy to deduce from his normal condition the accidents and incidents which could eventually change his life.

The Saturnian is predisposed to a number of physical and psychological disorders.

Physical Disorders
The Saturnian's health is unstable, maintained only by the disciplined life he leads and the restrictions to which he submits himself voluntarily. He is thin and wasted – really only skin and bone. His muscles are poorly developed and he has little inclination for physical exercise, a proclivity reinforced by his clumsiness. The Saturnian is one who fails to burn up his toxins or excrete unwanted metabolites. He lives with the minimum of physical exertion – Saturnians owe their longevity to a deep-rooted instinct of economy, which saves the carefully-guarded breath of life. Elimination of toxins is poor, and the resulting maladies include arterial hypertension, arteriosclerosis, biliary and renal stones. They live to a great age, even though prone to early senility, sustained by a miserable organic balance, for they spend little energy and are thus able to keep going to the last possible minute.

person who has been transmuted – markedly altered – by his illness. But not all diseases are microbial, and the toxins which attack an individual are often of psychological origin – toxins of worry, toxins of grief; moral toxins which shatter a person and alter his physical appearance to the point of complete change. Nevertheless, the subject, if he is a Saturn, will remain a Saturn, and you will simply witness an exaggerated development of certain characteristic elements. These are manifest, not by the appearance of new signs, but by a deeper and more marked expression of the usual signs of nervous disorder – sensory, motor and psychological. These are simply a paroxysm, an increase of the usual characteristics of the Saturnian. This results in a new 'significant expression', a new sign which appears, showing the overwhelming of the subject, his 'transmutation', for which the deep reasons and the remedies can be known simultaneously.

Morbid Predispositions
You are now familiar with the Saturnian at rest and in action, his intellectual resources and his

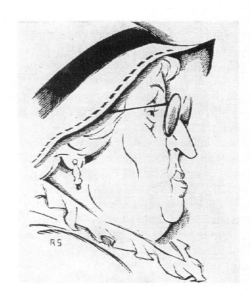

Psychological Disorders

The Saturnian is melancholic. His black, bilious moods are insupportable, whilst his intransigent pride gradually estranges him from his friends; his natural suspiciousness increases to paranoia, and his principle of economy becomes so strict that it leads him progressively to sordid avarice. His inveterate pessimism develops into a growing tendency to obsession.

Such are the mental maladies of the Saturnian: egoism, obsession, avarice, neurasthenia. They are not inevitable. A Saturn subject does not have to undergo these vexing transformations, even though he is 'naturally predisposed' to them. Can this tendency be countered? Certainly it can, because it is the result of organic deficiency. Remember that the Saturnian absorbs everything that comes within his range, retaining everything and rejecting virtually nothing. He is a deeply toxic individual, poisoned as much by autogenous toxins as by those of extrinsic origin, whether microbial or moral. Mental 'toxins' (for example, the hurtful behaviour of others) may appear to him to come from outside himself, but they are often provoked by an exaggeration of his own behaviour, such as his critical assessment of others, his natural suspicion, or his pessimistic interpretation of the slightest word or gesture. The Saturnian often suffers from delusions of persecution, and finds himself bereft of all religious feelings, involved though he be in the study of exegesis. At once sceptical and credulous, and further unbalanced by his researches into occultism, he seeks deliverance in death, even though he dreads it, and kills himself.

Sometimes, in the hope of escaping from the ideas which obsess him, the Saturnian flings himself wholeheartedly into religion, and gradually adopts total mysticism. His unwavering devotion allows of no respite. The religious Saturnian woman is the grand inquisitress of the habits of her companions. Her freely-voiced judgements, delivered in sententious language, strike the young women around her like a series of blows, inconsiderate and unanswerable. Her boundless pride does not stop short of slander.

The bad Saturnian woman fits well into the mediaeval concept of a witch. She is a vicious person, avaricious, spiteful and vindictive, taciturn and disquieting. She looks enviously around her; disagreeable and quarrelsome, she particularly seeks to upset lovers, of whose happiness she is jealous. Slander and libel are her stock-in-trade, the anonymous letter her favourite weapon.

Modifications of the Type

Physical and mental disorders cannot develop without profoundly altering the organic system of the Saturnian. The type of an individual is an impression, from within outwards, which relates to the behaviour of the subject. Physical or psychological disturbance of behaviour results in a changed appearance. Consider these signs:

The face is even thinner, the cheeks hollow, the cheek-bones more prominent. The forehead is creased with numerous tormented lines. The complexion is leaden or sometimes olive-coloured, the small black eyes are deeply set within the orbits, the gaze is dark and anxious. He is weak-sighted, with increased myopia. His body often exudes an unpleasant odour. His feeble legs have numerous varicose veins, and sometimes varicose ulcers.

In the field of mental illness, sick Saturnians are ceaselessly agitated by anxiety, dread, suspicion, distrust and envy. They spy on others and lay traps for them. Burning avarice makes them cruel usurers. Human relationships mean little to them; they care not for wife or child; the love of possessions alone dominates their actions. Slanderers, blackmailers, traitors, they are cowardly and full of hatred. Tormented by mistrust and fear, they carefully check the locks on all the doors and windows of the house before retiring, and then, unable to rest at night, tremble at the slightest sound or wake with a jerk, a prey to sudden terrors. The 'moral maladies' of the Saturnian are egoism and avarice, which lead him without his realising it to neurasthenia or insanity.

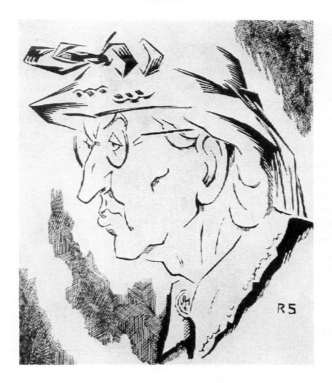

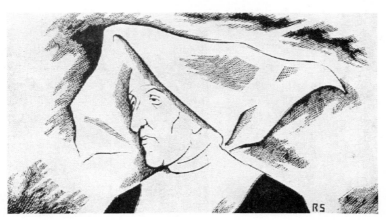

Such a state of affairs can be treated, although there is no remedy which will at once remove all the vexing propensities of the Saturnian. If such a therapy did exist, which could transform into perfect people those unfortunate wretches whose life seems to be dedicated to evil-doing, society would be greatly to blame for not using it. Nevertheless, a physician can treat the temperament to prevent or postpone some negative development which is foreseeable but not inevitable. Such an outcome can be predicted by signs which arise in the sick person, and these signs correspond to remedies which homoeopaths know well and use in daily practice.

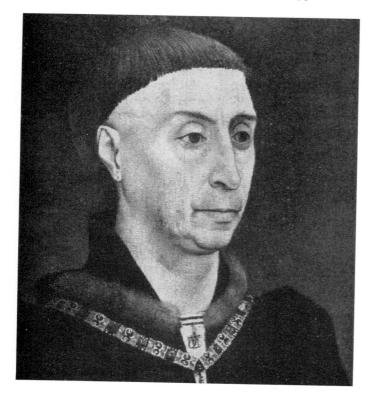

Roger van der Weyden, *Philip the Good*, fragment (Antwerp Museum, photo Bulloz)

Van der Goes, *Portrait of a Monk*, fragment (New York, photo Bulloz)

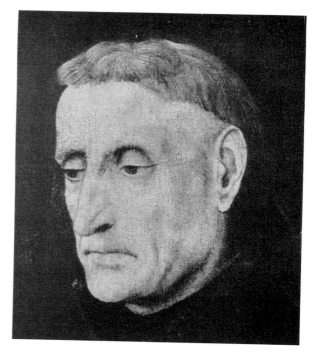

TREATMENT

It is extremely rare nowadays to come upon a pure Saturnian, but amongst the complex typologies seen in our patients, some will show Saturnian characteristics in their metatypes. It is useful to study in advance the remedies which act on them, in order to be able to correct, if only slightly, their adverse tendencies.

Basic Remedies

The basic remedies used by homoeopaths are those best adapted to the temperament of the subject; when used correctly they can powerfully alter the situation. They are best given in high potency and must not be repeated often.

The materia medica offers two principal remedies for the Saturnian – Sepia and Thuja. It is rare to find a Saturnian subject who does not need one of these remedies at some time during his life. This can be shown by recalling their chief indications.

Sepia

Sadness and prostration. Ali that this patient experiences is a darkness of the soul. Think of the black fluid which the squid discharges in moments of danger. Just as the cephalopod darkens the water around her, so the Sepia subject seems to be surrounded by gloom and obscurity. He sees the black side of everything, is dejected and depressed, miserable and interested in nothing.

Physically and mentally fatigued, he is misanthropic and taciturn, irritable and glum. When questioned, he replies briefly in monosyllables. He cannot be distracted, or share in any joy, but spends his time dispensing darkness. He no longer takes any interest in his usual occupations, work, business or family. All are one to him. He wants no distraction and seeks no pleasure. He is unsociable and likes to go for long walks by himself, which may for a while restore his equilibrium by improving his circulation. He is thoroughly disagreeable in company, easily vexed and aggravated. Irritated by others, and also by himself, he seeks for solitude.

A sensation characteristic of Sepia is intense and continuous pressure felt in the lower part of the abdomen, forcing the patient to cross his legs and bend forward when sitting. This is a favourite position of Sepia. Even the expression of the Sepia patient is typically Saturnian – heavy drooping eyelids, eyes half closed. Finally, the Sepia patient is liverish, with constipation, difficult and offensive urination, lumbosacral pain. He is always tired and run-down.

Thuja

Sadness and ill-humour are the dominant mental qualities of Thuja; but most characteristic of all is the tendency to obsession.

The materia medica contains numerous modalities relating to obsession. The patient believes someone is following him, or walking beside him in the road, that his body is a brittle glass vessel which the smallest shock could shatter, that he feels a live animal moving around in his belly . . . All these hallucinations are found in Thuja, but most important is the tendency to obsession itself. If the patient has worries, even small ones, he thinks about them constantly, for hours and days. One obsession is quickly followed by another, which may be similar, but equally unimportant – a forgotten letter, a broken glass, a misplaced object.

This tendency to obsession is usually accompanied by a feeling of weakness in the legs, which causes staggering. Sadness, constant futile preoccupations and unsteady gait are important symptoms of Thuja that are also found in the behaviour of the Saturnian. Add to this his difficulty in getting to sleep, and waking at 4 a.m., constipation, rheumatic deformities, a dirty greasy slimy skin, unpleasant body odour, marked venous distension, varicosities on the side of the nose. These are all signs frequently found in the Saturnian.

Closer study of these two remedies allows them to be differentiated easily, because their dominant characteristics are very different. A patient may need Sepia or Thuja, but not both, although both are the principal remedies for

Saturnians. The distinction is not only due to the fact that they show different symptoms, but that different causes will have led to the appearance of these symptoms.

Sepia always appears against a tuberculinic background. Venous congestion leading to portal hypertension is the essential cause of certain symptoms described, such as hepatic disorder and a yellowish saddle-mark across the nose. When the patient is carefully examined, the functional and objective signs of tuberculinism will easily be found, whether in the thoracic and pulmonary area or in the iris. Sepia will bring about amelioration in the patient, but may not be sufficient to cure. The prescription of diluted tuberculins, with suitable drainage, should bring about the desired result.

Thuja is more likely to be needed in subjects who have undergone repeated vaccinations, or who have suffered from genital disorders, such as a gonococcal discharge. Gonorrhoea should not be thought of as an acute disease which is cured when the discharge is checked by suppressive methods. It is true that the gonococcus has gone but its toxin remains, and little by little, under its influence the patient undergoes a slow transformation, a real psychological and organic change.

The essential characteristic of Thuja lies in its extraordinary tendency to promote growths of an unpleasant nature, as if the organism sought to deliver itself from its toxins by throwing out a piece of itself and thereby limiting the damage. The classical evolution of the Thuja subject is always the same. First, the production of benign tumours – warts, papillomas, lipomas, etc; significant events which should be considered as alarm signals, not to be neglected. Later malignant tumours may appear which lead to death, as the vital force of the subject is progressively used up.

Auxiliary Remedies

Hypertensive and arteriosclerotic disease, both common in Saturnians, demand the use of Baryta Carb. and Plumbum. Writers in the Middle Ages pointed out the close correspondence between Saturn and Lead. 'Spirit of Saturn' (lead acetate) was often used in mediaeval times. Baryta Carb. is well known for slowness of movement, as well as for another key symptom – men with mask-like rigid faces and women with masculine faces. Nor must Aurum be neglected; it is valuable in aortitis, and in that mental disorder whose progressive deterioration leads to suicide in the obsessional patient. This subject often suffers from a hereditary or acquired syphilitic taint, and has a fluoric constitution.

Biliary and renal calculi suggest certain remedies. The practitioner who needs to ensure the elimination of toxins will think of Berberis, Nux Vomica and Solidago Virga. Rheumatic manifestations will respond to Rhus Tox., Natrum Sulph. and Causticum. Debilitated states, so common in the Saturnian, will usually respond to Sepia or Thuja, although the symptoms may present other pictures.

Gelsemium is a remarkable remedy. The patient appears stupid and self-absorbed, unable to concentrate his thoughts or take a decision. He has difficulty in keeping his eyes open – the lids are so heavy and drooping, like those of Sepia and Causticum. He has lost all self-confidence and cannot speak in public, even when he has been accustomed to doing so all his life. His legs are weak and trembling.

Baryta Carbonica is not only a remedy for hypertension. It is very suitable for the depleted Saturnian who suspects everyone, fears everything and does not want to meet strangers. His memory is weak, he loses himself in streets which he knows perfectly well, he forgets everything, including the common names of things and especially proper names. We knew an unfortunate old gentleman who in his latter years constantly searched the telephone directory for the names of his friends.

Causticum also suits elderly Saturnians who show the following curious characteristic. During the day they are tranquil, albeit authoritarian and interfering, but when night falls they are possessed by anxiety; they get up and walk about all night long, prey to a delirium that is

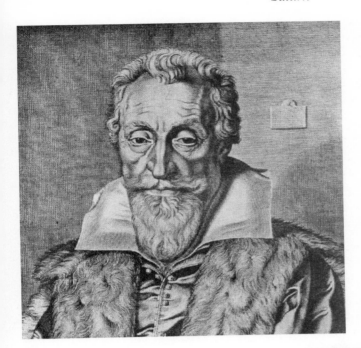

Above:
M. Lasné, *Nicolas Bruart de Sillery*

Below Left:
Rumpf, *Henrich Heine*, fragment (photo GG)

Below Right:
Simon Marmion, *Philip the Bold*, fragment (Versailles Museum, photo Giraudon)

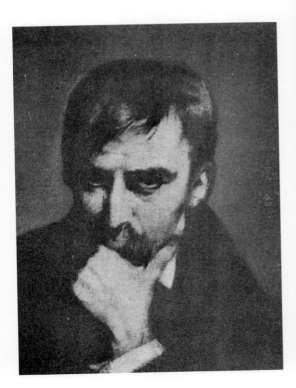

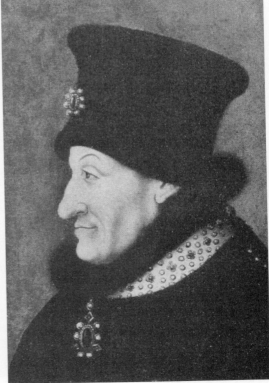

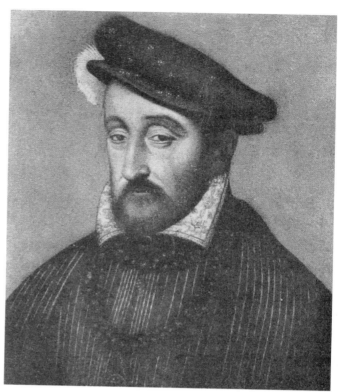

Above:
Francois Clouet, *Henri II* (Louvre Museum, photo LL)

Below Left:
E. Suau, *Edouard Branly*, fragment (photo Braun)

Below Right:
Anonymous Artist, *William Tyndale*, (photo B. Matthews)

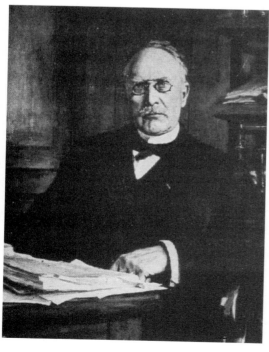

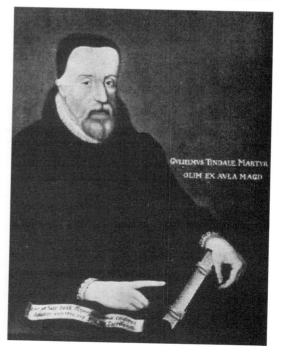

not violent but very agitated. We remember a patient of seventy-two, known all his life for high moral courage and great culture, who greeted us in the morning exhausted, as he said, by a long march. He did not remember that he had walked about all night, in and out of his apartment and up and down the stairs, flanked by his nurse who prevented him from ringing his neighbours' bells or going out into the road.

Finally, do not forget to use the prime remedy for auto-intoxication, Sulphur. The indications for this will usually appear when the Saturnian begins to deteriorate.

Never forget that homoeopathy is more than symptomatic treatment – a therapy determined by the symptoms which the patient presents – but that it is also a method of dealing with the true cause of all disease. Nosodes must be used according to their indications: Psorinum, Medorrhinum, Syphilinum and the potentized Tuberculins.

Saturnian illness is an extended chronic process, and treatment must be persevered with for a long time in order to obtain results.

Life Style

By life style we mean more than just a diet which any doctor could prescribe for his patient after taking account of the facts. The Saturnian needs advice about his whole way of life. First, he must be brought out of the physical inertia into which he has sunk, and be encouraged to exercise. It is unlikely that he could be persuaded to take up a sport, as he feels too feeble and debilitated, and his pride would be hurt if he were clumsy; but at least he should be advised to devote a short period every morning to physical exercises, to give him the suppleness he lacks, and he should walk for an hour every day.

Another point must be mentioned. Saturnians have antipathies of which one needs to be aware, in order to avert the antagonisms that can arise in their presence. Saturn is totally incompatible with Venus. The Saturnian woman hates the Venusian woman and will have nothing to do with her, even at a social gathering. Saturn does not get on well with Mars, whose violence and authoritarianism annoy him, nor yet with Jupiter, whose cheerfulness exasperates him. Mercury, on the other hand, is acceptable, because Saturn appreciates his gentleness and his ingenious mind.

The complementary type of Saturn is Earth, and more especially Cybele (Earth, Mercury) who by her smiling friendliness neutralises his tyranny.

In conclusion, we repeat: Saturn was born feeble and dies an octogenarian, having dragged his obsessions and his sadness through a life of misery . . . and having meanwhile bored others to death.

SATURN: THE REMEDIES

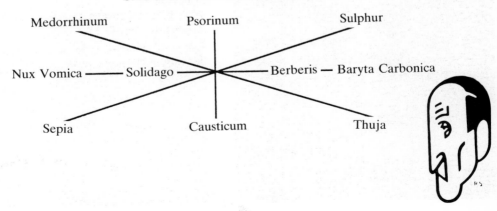

Medorrhinum — Psorinum — Sulphur

Nux Vomica —— Solidago —— Berberis — Baryta Carbonica

Sepia — Causticum — Thuja

6

Apollo

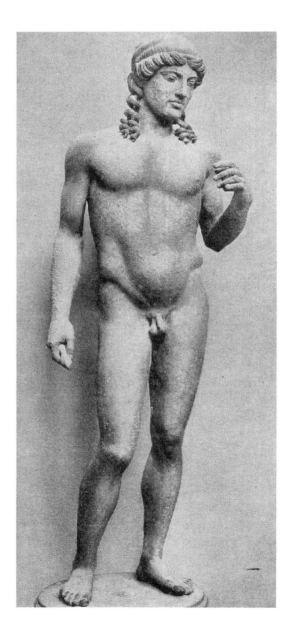

Apolonon the Cleanser, the Liberator. Phoebus Apollo was originally the god of the silver bow who aimed his arrows far and wide. He personified the free man, the hunter who lived off Nature without regard for laws. Later he would become Helios, god of the sun's golden disc.

He is still god of the lyre, god of song, of the bow, of the Muse and of Poetry, of everything that lets a living being pour out his heart into the world. Slim and supple, vibrating like the strings of his lyre, this is a lyrical feminine god, a god of rhythm and beauty. Apollo is the man of freedom who opposes the man of authority: Prometheus who stole fire from Jupiter and gave it to men, the rebellious perverse spirit who disturbs the world order with tumultuous heart and cries of passion. Apollonians are great lyricists, like Lord Byron and Chopin; sublime artists, like Raphael. The figure of Christ, as represented by numerous artists, shows all the characteristics of an Apollonian.

DOMINANT CHARACTERISTICS

Tall stature.
Nonchalant attitude.
Graceful, supple.
Love of beauty; indolent and self-regarding; lacking in common sense.

School of Praxiteles, *Apollo with Lyre* (Naples Museum, photo Bulloz)

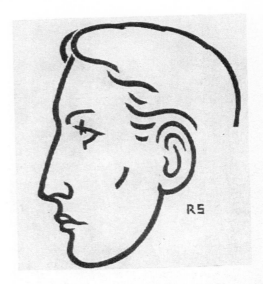

DESCRIPTION

Tall stature (1.70–1.80m in a man). Cool manner, indolent but graceful. Lithe, supple gait. Slow harmonious gestures. Moderately elongated skull (sub-dolicocephalic). Well-formed, medium-sized, slightly aquiline nose. Small well-shaped mouth. Light chestnut-coloured hair. Well-marked eyebrows. Large, widely open, light-coloured eyes. Pink complexion. Slim bust and small chest.

The arms are lightly muscled but graceful. The hands are long, with tapering fingers. The legs are long and flexible. The feet are long, slim and arched.

MORPHOLOGY

Static

Although less tall than the Marsian and the Saturnian, the Apollonian is of slightly more than medium height. Slim and elegant, the Apollonian subject is always well-proportioned. His aristocratic features are calm and thoughtful, neither sad nor cheerful, but rather grave and serene. He rarely laughs, but will smile benevolently out of politeness.

His face is oval, olive-shaped. His skull is slightly lengthened, but the vault is domed like a cupola. His rather prominent forehead rises to a dome; the skin is flexible, without permanent wrinkles, and he is often prematurely bald. His hair is long, soft and fine, of a pale red or light brown colour – 'ripe chestnut' to use a mediaeval expression. His eyebrows are moderately arched, always well-shaped and of the same colour as his hair. The upper eyelid droops slightly at its external canthus.

His eyes are saffron-coloured, spangled with points of light, gentle and serious in expression, wide open and framed by thin lids furnished with long eyelashes. The gaze is direct but not aggressive; masterful and fascinating, it seems illuminated by an inner radiance, speaking of distant, generous and unselfish thought. Elsewhere the eyes of the Apollonian have been described as 'luminous', but this term is open to equivocation. Unquestionably, Apollonian eyes are both light and clear, and their limpidity arises either from a special physical condition, a kind of transparency, or more probably from an interior purity, the reflection of a spirit enamoured of beauty and noble thoughts.

We describe the eyes of the Apollonian as clear and limpid, but wonder whether the character of Apollo, as learned from his expression, does not show a contradiction between the serenity of the face and a certain interior sadness, without bitterness, seen in the clear but melancholy eye – luminous only because of the quality of the internal being it reflects. It is as if the Apollonian was aware of his own weakness, and accepted the fate with which he was burdened.

The slightly aquiline nose is slim and of perfect contour, finely drawn without exaggeration or prominence. Its tip is firm and does not turn up or down; the nostrils are neat and pretty. The small mouth is perfectly shaped. The lips are tinted, firm and without thickness; the upper lip extends slightly beyond the lower. The chin is slender, of medium size, with a firm, rounded outline, and projects forward slightly. The beard is not heavy, but well-established and curly. Cheekbones and jawbones never project. The ears are small, nicely whorled, with slender

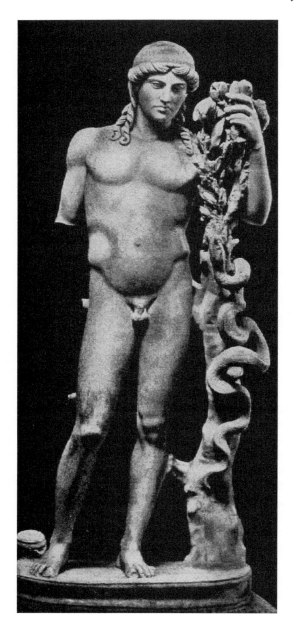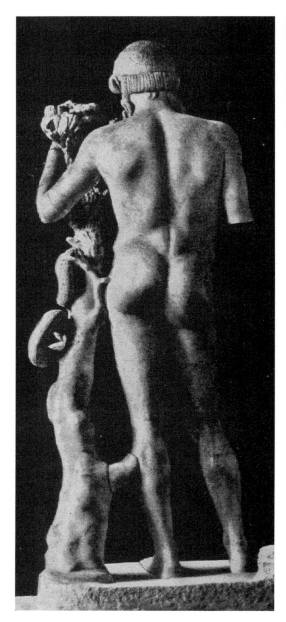

The Apollo of Mantua, detail (Mantua, Ducal
Palace, photo Premi (Dedalo))

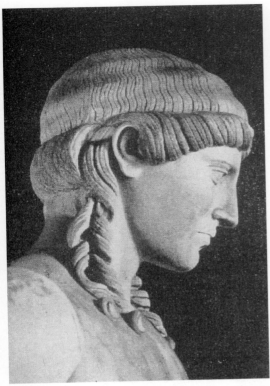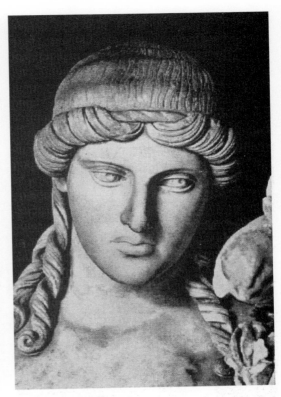

The Apollo of Mantua, (Mantua, Ducal Palace,
photo Premi (Dedalo))

lobes which are partially detached. The complexion is often pink, sometimes pale with patches of deeper colour here and there. The head is held erect without stiffness. The well-shaped slender neck is long, without looking thin. In women it is gracefully curved and covered with curly ringlets.

The body of an Apollonian is always well-constructed and well-proportioned. The bust is slim, the chest narrow; in women the breasts are small, firm, neatly rounded, with almost invisible nipples. All the muscles are fine and delicate. The back is flexible, the vertebrae not prominent, the shoulders sloping, thin and straight. The arms are long, with slender graceful muscles and a smooth, fine skin. The hands are supple and soft, with long smooth tapering fingers. The palms and digits are of equal length. The loins are arched; the thighs, smoothly muscled, are not massive; the legs are long and flexible; the knee-joints, not prominent, appear to lack muscle. The calves also are not muscular, but the legs are well-proportioned and of a beautiful shape. The feet are long, thin and arched.

Kinetic

The Apollonian's posture is elegant and graceful; his manner is cool and indolent. He does not seem to join in with the life of those around him, despite the internal excitement which constantly shakes him. The calmness with which he faces the world is only superficial, the result of a discipline self-imposed since youth. But in practice external happenings do not bother him much, since he feels himself superior to them. The gait of an Apollonian is always flexible, supple and graceful, rhythmic and harmonious.

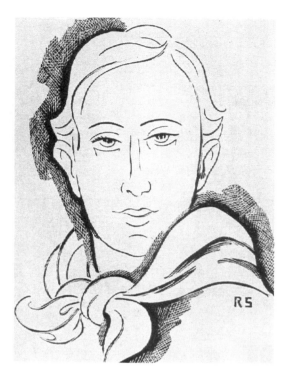

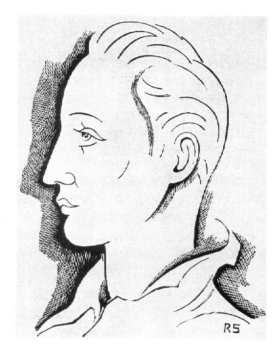

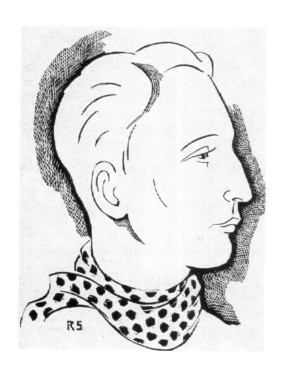

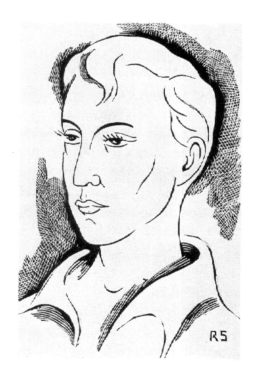

His gestures are smooth and unhurried. The dignity and controlled ease of his movements is astonishingly constant. Superficial minds mistakenly attribute to the Apollonian a deliberate pose with studied effects. But in fact, when he is with intimate friends, or alone, he still moves in the same easy confident way. It is a sign of his temperament and the reserve which he has imposed upon himself since childhood, leading to self-mastery and concentration.

Reinforced by the high opinion he has of his own personality, this admirable self-discipline gives him real distinction and constitutes a powerful charm.

His voice is soft and low, pure, serious, slow, harmonious and penetrating.

FUNCTIONS OF THE TYPE

Mind

Imagination is the dominant faculty of the Apollonian. It enables him to construct an inner life, hidden in the depths of his being; it also lights the flame which will rapidly destroy him if he cannot bring it to the surface. Nervous and highly-strung, he is a prey to thoughts and feelings; sanguine, he projects them into the world. He expresses himself personally, and rarely quotes anyone else. If he is an introvert he dreams his dreams; if extroverted, he tells them in a way that gains admiration.

If his forehead is wide, his intelligence is strongly poetic. If on the other hand he has a narrow skull, he is a bird-brain who can be trapped by romantic imaginings. He is a butterfly, attracted by light, throwing itself against a window-pane that it has not seen.

The Apollonian has marked artistic tendencies and loves order; ugliness repels him, to the extent that he cannot bear it in his servants, and shuns sick people and those unfortunates whose physical malformations make him feel really ill. He is of superior intelligence, understands everything, and is a good judge of art – if we are speaking of a fugue, a fresco, a monument or a tragedy. But often he practises no form of creative art himself, unless Art is a necessity for his self-expression. Then he works hard but is never satisfied with what he has produced, because it is so far from corresponding with the interior vision that illuminates him. His life is given to his ideal, as a woman gives hers to her child; and it becomes a ferment of beauty and lyricism, or of rebellion. The Apollonian may be a poet or an artist, he is always enthusiastic and passionate. His vast intelligence allows him to encompass everything, to conceive of everything, to grasp the whole in a single intuitive moment.

Apollonians love literature and the arts, and cultivate them successfully. They prefer music of a serious and religious nature. They also have a remarkable aptitude for the occult sciences, and possess the sacred fire of divination which may inspire them to prophesy. Endowed with singular clairvoyance, they can foresee revolutions and other great changes, even though they do not always profit from the knowledge.

The Apollonian sees everything clearly except himself, and cannot understand the reasons for his misfortunes which are, like his successes, tremendous.

Character

Ardent and passionate by nature, the Apollonian is mobile, capricious, hard to please, finicky, ironical and mocking. His power of psychological penetration shows him the imperfections of others. He is polite without familiarity, tending to keep people at a distance.

He has no patience with indelicacy or untruth and speaks his mind readily to dishonest people. Should a social lie seem necessary he prefers to keep silent, and he never flatters. His opinion of himself matters much more to him than that of others, and he will sacrifice everything to his own reputation.

His pride is internal, arising from an idealised conception which he is continuously writing into the drama of his life, without ever tiring of doing so. He has a stimulating effect on his companions, who respect and admire him without really understanding him, and often mistake for overweening pride that which is no more than an unattainable quest for perfection.

Sober, not very sensual, shunning excess and only giving the barest attention to bodily necessities, the Apollonian does nevertheless take an interest in his appearance. However simple his private life, he will adorn himself with sumptuous luxury when he appears in public. He was born to be rich; poverty is incompatible with this too-perfectly evolved individual who cannot cope with the hard facts of life. If these should overcome him, he will die after a short illness.

The Apollonian likes to shine and to protect, but he needs a comfortable background and preferably a harmonious, artistic environment. If he is rich he spends his money well and in good taste, only buying the best works of art. He knows how to create his surroundings, and only consorts with worthwhile people.

It lies within the destiny of Apollonians to be loaded with honours, even when they have started from a lowly position. They are also subject to strange changes of fortune, and their astonishing rise is often followed by a resounding fall. Men of destiny, as they believe themselves to be, they bear these reverses with admirable strength of mind, and never despair. Those less favoured by luck, birth or riches see themselves as unknown geniuses. In spite of any number of disappointments they will persevere in careers that bring them nothing but scorn.

The Apollonian needs light; the sun is for him a powerful restorer. He cannot bear dull, gloomy weather, which makes him profoundly sad. Sometimes his aversion for darkness, which he peoples with ghosts, is so great that he cannot sleep at night unless the light is on.

Of a feminine temperament, and not sexually over-active, he loves from vanity, wishing to attract the interest of an admired and sought-after object. He loves poetically, illustrating the model of a grand passion. He may also love perversely, seeking to suffer and to inflict suffering, simply for the pleasure of thrilling and being thrilled, in a ceaseless search for voluptuous sensation. But his eagerness and desire to please stop short of total commitment.

The object he loves above all is himself. Never tired of admiring his own image, he spends the best part of his life in seeking to project it to the greatest advantage – a proud self-lover who, like Narcissus, drowns in his own reflection. Alternatively, he can be the one who sacrifices himself for a magnificent ideal. Such a man is regarded as inspired, firing others with compassionate and uplifting thoughts.

THE APOLLONIAN WOMAN

Charming and delicate, well-mannered and usually well-educated, the Apollonian woman is always young – there is no time in her life for growing old. She is born to luxury and is not armed for battle. Art is her aim, her life, her *raison d'être* – she herself is a work of art, and knows it, and admires herself as such.

She has a horror of figures and does not know how to count. Imagination grips her and she lives in a sort of dream, wholly concerned with the impression, deep or shallow, that she can produce on others. She lives in the hope of achieving what she believes to be her right, and to dominate and shine.

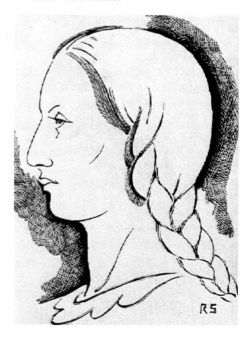

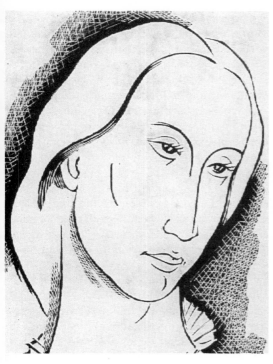

If she is a superior person she will devote herself to a man who occupies a high position, making him a dutiful wife, careful of her reputation and all the proprieties. She would be a marvellous companion for a statesman or diplomat, but could not accommodate herself to a bourgeois existence without a future.

If she is an inferior person she will make unjustified pretensions. These will be the more preposterous because, as a false Muse and false devotee, hateful, demanding, proud and lacking genius, she appears as a caricature of the true Apollonian. The one prefers obscurity to compromise and would live in hiding rather than submit to servility; the other makes a bid to achieve notoriety by bizarre and risky means.

The Apollonian woman loves dressing up. She adores jewels, pearls, sapphires and fine silks; she cannot pass a mirror without stopping for the pleasure of admiring herself. She is subject to migraine and debility, leading to exhaustion and feverish episodes. She should beware of using perfumes (which she adores) that titillate the sense of smell. Nor can she

resist the temptations of morphine, ether and cocaine; these enable her to escape from the heavy realities of life but use up her cerebral energy. Constantly seeking spurious energy from new addictions, she will terminate tragically in madness or death.

Intoxication with drugs and intoxication with pleasure are as dangerous to the male Apollonian as to the female. Both thrill to every luxury that tempts them, just as both shudder from all the vulgarities that shock them.

Life Style

The Apollonian is a poet and a dreamer, and rather lazy, since he is lymphatic and soft. Still, he cannot resist the pleasure of going to see beautiful flowers and beautiful places – you, the physician, will always be popular if you advise him to go to mountain resorts or balmy climates where he is able to bask in the air and sunshine that are so necessary to his life. His pleasure will be turned into intoxicating joy if his surroundings include compatible people and artistic entertainment.

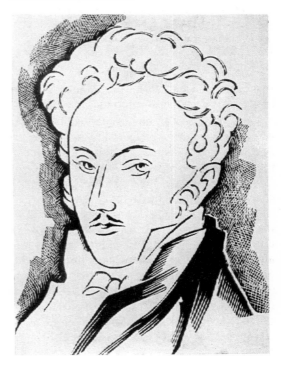

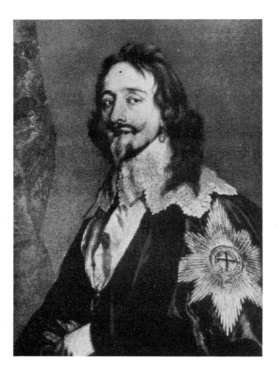

Sir Peter Lely, *King Charles I of England*, fragment (Dresden Museum, photo Giraudon)

DISEASES AND REMEDIES OF THE APOLLONIAN

The characteristics of an Apollonian will be modified by the constitution to which he belongs. One fact is immediately evident: the Apollonian is never a Carbonic. He is usually Phosphoric, sometimes Fluoric, and more generally Phospho-Fluoric.

Carbonic Constitution

The Carbonic is seen in the rigidity of his build; the regularity which is a constant feature of his unhurried discipline; his endurance and his strength. None of these is ever found in the Apollonian, whose physical and dynamic characteristics are essentially different from those of the Carbonic. On the other hand, the usual manifestations of the Phosphoric constitution are analogous to those of the Apollonian.

Phosphoric Constitution

The Phosphoric is a delicate, slim individual, tall and spare with an elegant gait and gracious, usually harmonious gestures. He is elegant by nature, but having no solid foundations is also fragile and offers little resistance to adversity. His hypersensitive nature goes with a love of rhythm and beauty, and the search for perfection is the aim of his life.

Compare with this the physical and dynamic characteristics of the Apollonian, as already described. The analogy is striking, and could not be otherwise considering the morbid predispositions of the Apollonian on the one hand, and the major causes of the formation and development of the Phosphoric constitution on the other.

Fluoric Constitution

The Apollonian may be purely Fluoric, but we are more likely to meet with individuals of mixed constitution, Fluorico-Phosphoric, or Phospho-Fluoric; they are distinguished by their remarkable ability to gather from their surroundings everything that will single them out and help them to satisfy their ambitions. These are practical Apollonians who know how to profit by their gifts, to assure themselves of the position in life which they need to fulfil their desires and tastes. Unfortunately, the desire for profit will cause them to commit faults, especially the one with which they are always reproached – that of subordinating Art to speculation.

TRANSMUTATIONS OF THE APOLLONIAN

We have already described our concept of the favourable and unfavourable aspects of a Type. When the unfavourable signs are present, when the aptitudes are no longer used correctly for the normal development of the subject, then the typical signs are exaggerated. It is easy to recognise the transformation which has taken place, whatever name one chooses to give it – unlucky, mischievous or evil.

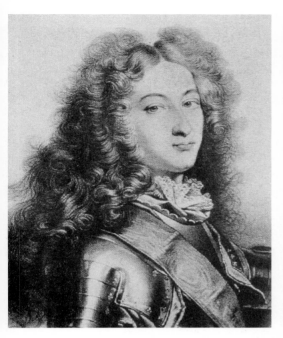

The Duke of Burgundy, father of Louis XV (photo Cie des Arts Photomécaniques)

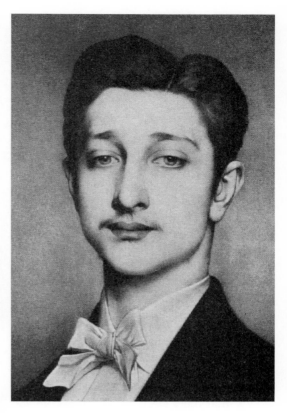

J. Lefevre, *The Prince Imperial*, fragment (Versailles Museum, photo Braun)

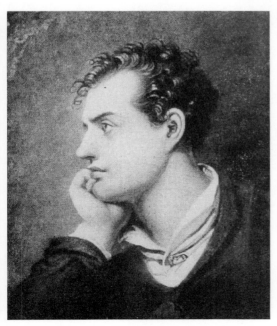

Lord Byron, fragment (photo Agence Photographique Française).

MORBID PREDISPOSITIONS

Physical Disorders

Physically the Apollonian is a creature of weak constitution and low resistance. If he avoids excess he does not become intoxicated in the usual sense of the term – that is, he does not absorb toxins; but in truth he is poisoned by the life he leads – a disturbed life ranging from enthusiasm to depression, from hyper-excitability to prostration. His weak spot is his respiratory system. Being disinclined for physical exercise, he neglects to breathe properly and too often his chest remains narrow and underdeveloped.

Everything for him is sacrificed to aesthetics. If he decides to walk on a beach so that all may

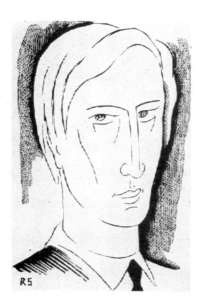

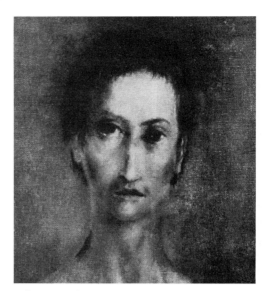

Leon Zack, *St. John the Baptist*, fragment
(photo 'Formes')

admire the perfection of his body, then he will not submit to any restrictive measures designed to preserve his health. Sometimes he will be overcome by sudden exhaustion, which will literally flatten him out for hours or days. Then his vitality will recover, only to relapse again after a short time. His nervous depressions and sudden weaknesses are accompanied by bouts of fever. These symptoms can last for quite a long time. If he loses weight, an X-ray may show a shadow at the apex of the lung. One thing is certain – the Apollonian is predisposed to tuberculosis, and is often suddenly carried off by what used to be called galloping consumption. In fact, the Apollonian is most often of the Phosphoric constitution, a tuberculinic whose organism rapidly burns out unless he adopts a regular life-style and puts himself under appropriate medical treatment.

Psychological Disorders

The serenity normally apparent in the bearing of an Apollonian gives way to confused agitation. He will use intrigue to achieve those things that he cannot obtain by his own efforts. The will to succeed – paramount in the Apollonian, especially when misdirected – acquires a sort of inhuman brutality, oblivious to right or wrong.

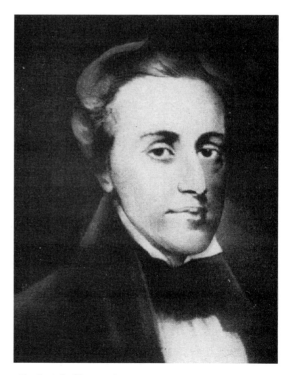

Frederick Chopin (photo Agence Photographique Française)

The Apollonian seeks for originality, and will construct curious paradoxes and stretch them to absurd lengths in order to attract attention. The Apollonian woman displays eccentric clothes in order to be noticed. Impelled by vanity she makes promises which she knows she cannot keep, boasting about influential connections and even about imaginary relatives with fictitious titles. To satisfy her thirst for notoriety she may go so far as to lie about herself and claim the role of villainess. Above all she must establish a personality of importance. In love, vanity is her guide. A famous man has the best chance of seducing her, whatever the reasons for his fame. Her passion is complicated by a deplorable factor – the desire to be noticed and to be different in an aesthetic sense from everyone else. Consequently the conditions of sexual intimacy must be bizarre in order to really please her.

There are Apollonians who dream, in their boundless ambition, of conquering the whole world and bringing it under their rule. Megalomania and paranoid delusions are often found amongst the Type.

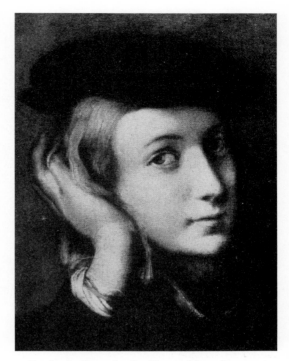

Raphael, *Portrait of a Young Man*, fragment (Louvre Museum, photo Bulloz)

Modifications of the Type

The following are the distinguishing features of the type. The upper part of the forehead is very prominent. Always anxious-looking, it is furrowed by horizontal lines. The short eyebrows are arched and dark. The sparkling eyes are set deep in their sockets, their gaze remote and haughty, reflecting the restless preoccupations passing through the mind. The eyelashes are short. The nose is neat, like that of a child, too small in proportion to the rest of the face. The upper lip almost completely covers the lower lip. The obstinate chin projects forward, and when it is large destroys the perfect oval of the face. The hair, truly blond, is curly.

The woman is in fact androgynous, with so little bosom that she could be said to have the chest of a boy. She is not animated by true sexuality and her amorous engagements are conducted in cold blood. But, magical actress that she is, her charms overwhelm those who

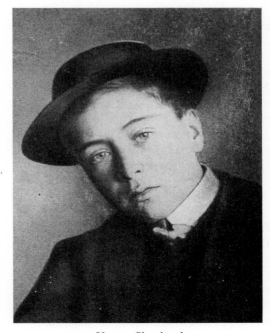

Young Shepherd

61

fall victim to them, so that they come to live in a world where fiction and fact are confused in an almost mad depravity.

TREATMENT

The Apollonian is always predisposed to tuberculosis and is often tuberculinic. The symptoms which he presents significantly express the remedies best suited to him. The major ones are described here.

Natrum Muriaticum

This is the great remedy for demineralisation. Various objective signs indicate that a patient is demineralised – white patches on the nails, dental caries, falling hair, and especially loss of weight.

When the loss of weight is slow and progressive, think of Natrum Mur. In spite of all his efforts, and those of his parents, the patient cannot gain weight. Indeed, he loses weight

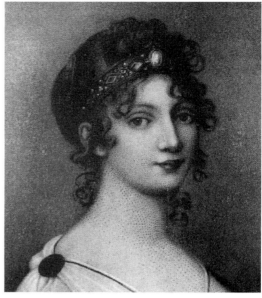

J. Grassi, *Queen Louise of Prussia*, fragment (Berlin, photo Stengel & Cie)

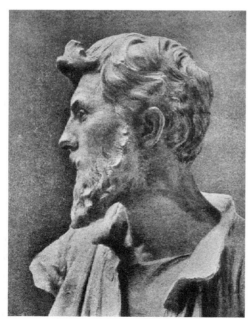

Edouard Lanteri, *The Labourer*, fragment (photo 'The Studio')

even whilst eating well. Tall, thin, with a spotty greasy face, he is constantly tired, more so in the morning than in the evening; he is weakest at 10 a.m. This physical weakness is accompanied by depression. The Natrum Mur. subject is sad, prefers to be alone, and strangely cannot bear to be consoled. If you talk gently to him, understanding his plight and seeking to help, he melts into tears. 'Weeps often at the slightest cause, and above all from consolation' is a characteristic of this remedy.

He is extraordinarily sensitive and lacks self-control. Thus he may fly into a rage for nothing, but more often shows his displeasure by sulking. The child who sits in a corner and sulks for no reason often needs Natrum Mur., particularly if he has a rash on his upper eyelids.

Sleep is often disturbed by nervous twitchings. Any unpleasant episode during the day will cause insomnia. One symptom unique to Natrum Mur. is that the subject dreams that robbers have come into the house and into his bedroom. A young boy or girl will frequently not reveal these dreams to their parents, who would be surprised to learn that their child never goes to bed without having made sure the doors are tightly shut, and inspecting all the corners of the room and looking under the bed.

The Natrum Mur. subject is incapable of prolonged intellectual work, because he suffers from violent headaches, either continuous or at periodic intervals of two or four days. There is an intense sensation of little hammer blows, or a feeling as if the head were about to explode. Overworked students and schoolchildren who suffer so badly from headaches that they have to give up their studies will generally be relieved by Natrum Mur. (Improvement from eating suggests Anacardium.)

To complete the picture, note that the Natrum Mur. subject is very sensitive to cold and catches colds easily: coryza, worse at 10 a.m., persistent tracheitis, palpitations, and incontinence of urine.

Insatiable thirst with desire for frequent large quantities of cold water, abnormal desire for salt, constipation with hard, dry stools which crumble at the edge of the anus, chronic lumbago worse on waking and needing a hard pillow in the small of the back (because it is always better for pressure), are also all characteristics of Natrum Mur. To these must be added some other interesting objective signs – herpes labialis, a fissure at the centre of the lower lip, and a 'geographical tongue'. Another curious fact is that the subject is unable to urinate while being watched; you can never persuade a Natrum Mur. child to urinate in your presence.

Natrum Mur. is the supreme remedy for an Apollonian who loses weight progressively after an emotional shock. The administration of a high potency of this remedy would seem instantly to reverse the process of decalcification. The patient gains weight in a manner which could not have been obtained by the oral or intravenous administration of massive doses of calcium salts.

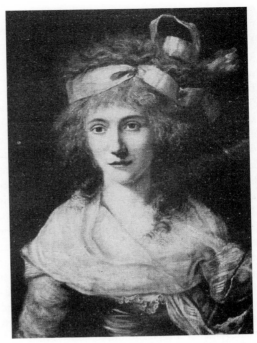

Théroigne de Méricourt, presumed portrait
(photo Bulloz)

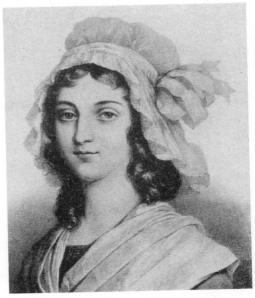

Charlotte Corday (photo Cie des Arts
Photomécaniques)

Ferrum Metallicum

This is an important remedy for the Apollonian. It relates to the nervous hypersensitivity of an Apollonian who, having become very irritable, has outbursts of anger or unheard-of violence from the smallest contradiction. Circulatory disorders are closely connected with nervous irritability. The subject will complain bitterly if all the mucous membranes – lips, gums and tongue – are extremely pale, and the face becomes suddenly flushed, attributing his condition entirely to emotional causes. But other signs indicate that the whole organism is affected: a violent throbbing headache, anorexia or voracious hunger, appetite for nothing but bread and butter, vomiting after midnight, diarrhoea which is more frequent at night, repeated epistaxes, amenorrhoea with vicarious haemorrhages (often epistaxis, sometimes haemoptysis). The weakness of the patient is demonstrated by his slow pulse, which accelerates at the least movement. Anaemia, weakness, circulatory disorders, nervous irritability, these are the attributes of the Ferrum subject, and they are also to be found in the Apollonian, who, it must not be forgotten, is always likely to have organic pathology.

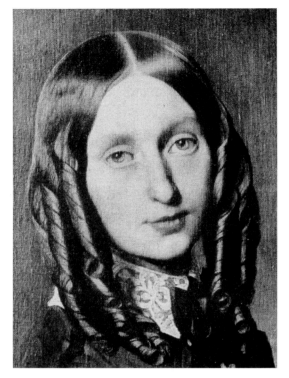

J.-D. Ingres, *Portrait of Mme Reiset*, fragment
(photo Bulloz)

Kali Carbonicum

This remedy shows another kind of anaemia. There are few or no vasomotor disorders, but instead a great weakness leading to total exhaustion. A keynote is that the subject cannot be left alone because he has an irrational fear of death, starts at the merest touch and jumps with fear at any physical contact. The smallest exertion provokes the appearance of copious cold sweats; thus during a meal you will see drops of sweat trickling down his lips and face. He has a phobia of draughts and is always shivering. One important characteristic must also not be forgotten – the tendency to oedema of the legs and especially of the eyelids. Swelling of the internal angle of the upper eyelid is a valuable sign in Kali Carb.

But Kali Carb. also shows signs of organic change: the cough, with characteristic expectoration of small, round grey masses, suddenly projected from the mouth without the patient being aware of it; asthma which reaches a crisis at 3 a.m.; sharp stabbing pains at the base of the right lung; considerable abdominal distension which develops as soon as the patient has taken any nourishment.

Iodum

This is a very different remedy. Ferrum and Kali Carb. correspond to two well-differentiated forms of anaemia, the one accompanying circulatory disorders, the other with localised oedema. Iodum is more like Natrum Mur. in that it has the same characteristic – 'loss of weight even while eating well' – but in this case the loss of weight, which may be considerable, takes place rapidly, despite the efforts of the patient, who is always hungry and never satisfied.

There is another interesting difference. Until now we have been considering anaemic and debilitated patients who wanted to be quiet. Iodum is constantly on the move and anxious, especially if a meal is delayed. He flies into a violent temper if he cannot eat as soon as he is hungry.

Another important feature is induration of the mammary, testicular and ovarian glands, as well as of the cervical, axillary, inguinal and mesenteric lymph nodes. The organism is attacked, the lymphatic tissue responds, glandular foci appear and crises of elimination follow – frothy, greasy morning diarrhoea, abundant and irritating, excoriating the skin and staining the clothes. It is important to remember that the Iodum patient is always too hot, and sometimes feverish.

Iodum is an excellent remedy for Basedow's disease, which is often found in the Apollonian.

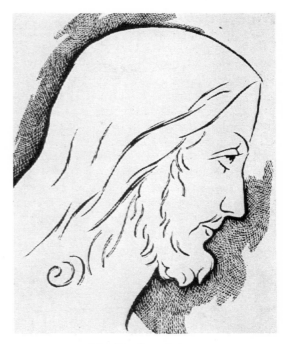

After Fra Bartolemeo

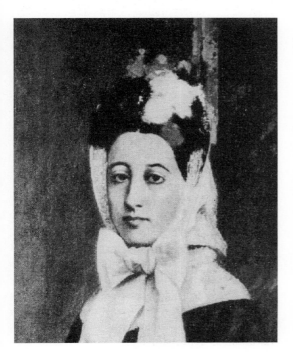

Degas, *Portrait of Mme Morbilli*, fragment (Jeu de Paume Museum, photo Formos)

Arsenicum Album

This remedy corresponds to a more serious condition whose essential feature is intermittence. In one moment, hour or day the patient feels well and can make great efforts; the next moment, hour or day he is debilitated and completely exhausted. Three important signs are: extreme agitation worse from 1–3 a.m. – an agitation which persists in spite of severe weakness, so that the patient demands at frequent intervals to be turned over in bed; anxiety with fear of death; burning pains as if from glowing coals, but always improved by heat.

Arsenicum is valuable in the treatment of chronic conditions which are none other than the defensive reaction of an organism which needs to eliminate toxins: burning leucorrhoea, which is irritating, yellowish, putrid and excoriating; and squamous eruptions, worse from the cold of winter, causing itching and burning which is relieved by very hot water. Lastly, the oedematous tendency of Kali Carb.

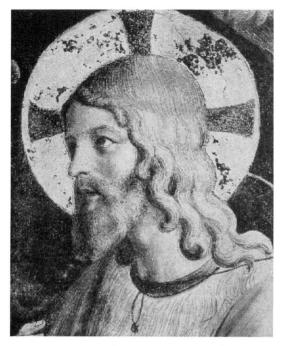

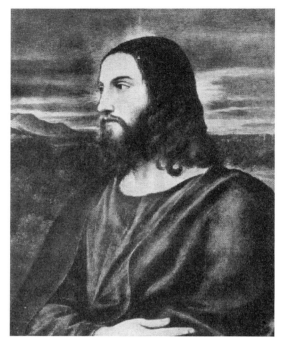

Fra Angelica, *Head of Christ*, fragment (Florence, St Mark Museum, photo Anderson-Giraudon)

Titian, *The Saviour*, fragment (Florence, Pitti Gallery, photo Anderson)

is even more marked in Arsenicum: swelling of the lower eyelids, oedema of the legs, and finally, anasarca.

Arsenicum is not only a remedy for chronic conditions. It also covers acute reactions presented by the patient: typhoid states with vomiting and diarrhoea; acute coryza, or hay fever; asthma, worse between midnight and 3 a.m.; pain in the upper third of the right lung.

Phosphorus

This remedy is only indicated in the Apollonian in severe acute disease: pulmonary congestion, generally with haemoptysis or acute gastro-enteritis. It is important not to repeat the remedy too often, to avoid complications. The Phosphorus cough is dry, irritating, painful and exhausting. The whole body shakes and the cough is accompanied by considerable oppression, with burning pains and a sensation of constriction in the chest. The patient must sit up in bed in order to expectorate, and the sputum

is purulent and bloodstained. Phosphorus is a good remedy for repeated haemoptyses, if it is not given too often. The patient is thirsty for cold water, which he then vomits.

The haemorrhages of Phosphorus are frequent and abundant, and typically remittant, whatever their location: epistaxis, haemoptysis, haematemesis, intestinal haemorrhage, haematuria. The slightest wound bleeds freely, and purpura and petechial haemorrhages are a further aspect of the haemorrhagic tendency of this subject.

The succession of remedies whose essential characteristics we have briefly outlined correspond closely to the unfolding stages usually associated with an untreated case of tuberculosis. These are: demineralisation (Natrum Mur.); nervous and circulatory disorders (Ferrum); depression with a tendency to oedema (Kali Carb.); glandular and lymphatic disorders (Iodum). Then the situation worsens and serious symptoms appear (Arsenicum or Phosphorus). Finally there is a diagnosis of organic damage with tissue destruction, which often calls for Stannum.

Treatment of the Apollonian offers a wider scope to those who understand it. Consider this subject, with his impressionability, his elation, his instability marked by alternations of enthusiasm and disappointment. Here are strong indications for Pulsatilla, especially if accompanied by venous congestion and bland yellow mucous secretions. Think also of Ignatia, called for in the depressions which may follow grief or frustration.

Pulsatilla

The keynote of Pulsatilla is the variability of symptoms presented by the patient. Everything alters, everything is changed: flitting pains, no two stools alike, an essentially unstable mood. Timid and fearful, he weeps for no reason but is easily consoled. This is the whingeing child who can laugh if you say something funny or distract him with a joke. Pulsatilla is easily discouraged and then becomes resigned, sad and melancholy. He cannot sleep at night, nor get up in the morning, and is more tired in the morning than at bedtime. Circulatory troubles are very marked: cyanosis of the extremities, a tendency to frostbite. The periods are late, scanty, more abundant by day, intermittent, and dark in colour. There is thick, ·milky, non-irritant leucorrhoea.

Other keynotes are the absence of thirst and the immediate aggravation when the patient goes from a cold atmosphere into a warm one. There is a tendency to congestion of the face and shivering without fever in a warm room. Venous engorgement and yellowish non-irritant mucous secretions (tears, coryza, expectoration, leucorrhoea) are important features of Pulsatilla, and their cause is often tuberculous in origin.

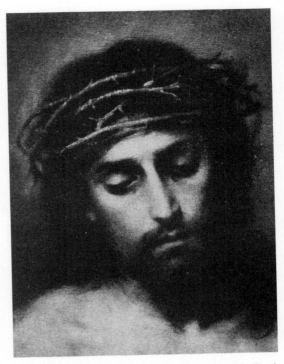

Murillo, *Ecce Homo*, fragment (Richmond, Cook Gallery, photo Anderson-Giraudon)

Ignatia

Like Pulsatilla, Ignatia shows a changeable mood. Its instability could be confused with that of Pulsatilla if there were not other marked differences between the two remedies. Here the patient is at one and the same time deeply sad and exuberantly happy. The symptoms of which she complains have two essential characteristics. These are: (i) a nervous depression which may be mental or emotional, and which is usually the result of grief or frustration; and (ii) the paradoxical nature of the symptoms – ringing in the ears relieved by music, sore throat which is better for swallowing, nausea which disappears on eating, gastric upsets which are worse when on a diet but which disappear after eating a rich meal, pain in the anus worse after a soft stool, haemorrhoids better for walking, diarrhoea from emotion or fear, a cough relieved by coughing, a spasmodic giggle on hearing sad news. Everything is contrary with Ignatia.

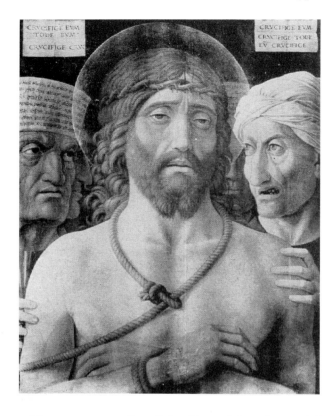

Mantegna, *The Mocking of Christ*, fragment. Note on the left the reasonable and logical Saturnian, on the right the brutal and vindictive Marsian. (Paris, Jacquemart-André Museum, photo Bulloz)

These two remedies, Pulsatilla and Ignatia, are both complementary to Natrum Mur., which is the principal agent for the repair of organic disease in the Phosphoric and the tuberculinic, where its action is needed for the recalcification of the patient.

After administration of a high potency of Natrum Mur. it would seem that the patient no longer loses calcium in his stools, the phosphaturia diminishes and the loss of weight slows down – indeed there may even be a weight gain. This recalcification will be even more marked if the patient is given the calcium salt appropriate to him – Calcarea Phosphorica. But it is not helpful to prescribe it in massive doses or intravenous injections; these only result in sudden, temporary ameliorations, after which all the alarming symptoms reappear, such as phosphaturia, constipation, and loss of weight. Calc. Phos. must be given homoeopathically – that is, not only in infinitesimal doses, but following the Law of Similars which rules all our prescribing.

Let us briefly recall the essential characteristics of Natrum Muriaticum:

Anaemic, restless, easily excited children who wake and cry at night.

Growing pains, with a sensation of stiffness in the neck and in the muscles.

Scholar's headache. As soon as he begins to study his head hurts.

All intellectual effort is difficult. The slightest thing frightens him. His complaints are worse for thinking about them.

Unusual hunger at 4 p.m.

Desire for salted and smoked meat.

Flaccid expanded belly. Umbilical colic.

Diarrhoea after cold drinks and during teething.

Early periods with violent backache. Leucorrhoea like egg-white.

We cannot terminate this therapeutic account without mentioning the importance for the Apollonian of prescriptions of Tuberculinum in potency, which, completing the action of the indicated homoeopathic remedies, constitutes both a true prophylactic therapy and an individualised immunotherapy.

'Providence', writes Ozanam, 'puts poets and artists in decadent societies, just as she puts birds' nests in ruins, to console them.' Painter or sculptor, poet or composer, the Apollonian is certainly 'he who sees and perceives', which is something many people do not know or fail to understand. Victim of a veritable Gehenna which tortures him painfully, the flame which animates him also devours him; but inspiration lights him on his way, his radiance nourishes and sustains him. If, at his best, he is the Inspired One, he is also the Shining One. He is in fact the Liberator and the Purifier who brings peace to men of good will.

Think of the appearance which painters of different epochs have given to Christ. The expression may vary according to the circumstances envisaged but the features are constant. It would seem that the artists have all followed the same plan and used the same set of reference points.

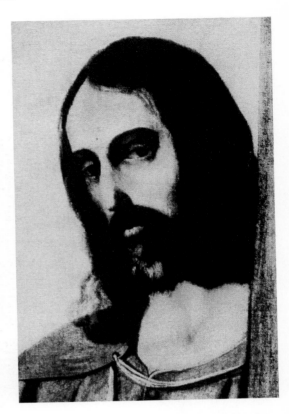

Zurbaran, *Scene from the Life of Jesus*, detail (Seville, Provincial Museum, photo Arxiu Mas)

APOLLO: THE REMEDIES

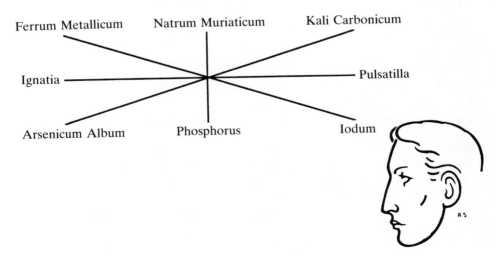

Ferrum Metallicum   Natrum Muriaticum   Kali Carbonicum

Ignatia ———————— Pulsatilla

Arsenicum Album   Phosphorus   Iodum

7

Venus

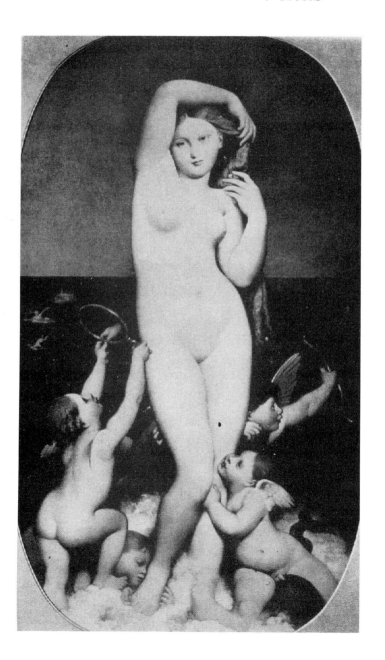

J.-D. Ingres
Venus Anadyomene (Chantilly,
Condé Museum, photo Bulloz)

The name of Venus should not bring forth images of a coarse or dissolute nature. To the Ancients, Venus incarnated the idea of love in its most noble and all-embracing sense. She united the goodness of the soul with the beauty of the body, and the grace she shows expresses the nobility of her sentiments.

Venus is the daughter of the wave, the goddess of beauty and love; a voluptuously pleasure-seeking lover of nature; the young girl in the picture by Greuze, caressing doves whilst thinking of the pleasures to come; the Madeleine of Guide, who expiates her past in dreaming of her heavenly future; Anne of Austria, who longs for Richelieu, even as she consoles herself with Mazarin; or Marie-Louise, determined to hold on to her imperial spouse Napoleon, even though he is also loved by Marie Walewska.

DOMINANT CHARACTERISTICS

Fairly tall.
Languid, indolent posture.
Leisurely, ponderous gait.
Peaceable character.
Very sociable, but lazy.

DESCRIPTION

Fairly tall (1.70–1.80m in a man). Relaxed, graceful, indolent pose. Leisurely, ponderous gait. Deliberate, all-embracing gestures. 'Egg-shaped' face. Smooth forehead, rounded skull. Beautifully-shaped nose, straight or slightly aquiline. Small, prettily-shaped mouth. Round plump chin, ornamented with a dimple.

Small, rather fleshy, nicely whorled ears. Black or brown hair, often curly. Well-marked, curving eyebrows. Soft brownish-black eyes. Smooth complexion.

Well-formed bust with a small waist and generous bosom. Plump arms without visible muscles, chubby hands and smooth fingers. Heavy fat legs without visible muscles, plump short feet.

MORPHOLOGY

Static

Two major features become obvious at the first examination: flowing curves and rounded limbs. The terms 'made to measure' or 'moulded' perfectly describe the Venusian appearance.

The head, small and regularly-featured, recalls that of a Greek statue, with full round cheeks (often thickened in old age) and no visible jawbone. The skull is rounded at the front and back and has no definite character, being either sub-brachycephalic or sub-dolicocephalic.

The face is egg-shaped. In youth the little end is the chin, but in old age the egg reverses and the chin becomes the base of the egg.

The forehead is short and rounded, never very prominent; it is usually smooth but heavily veined, and in states of emotion the venules

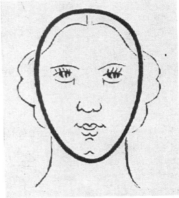

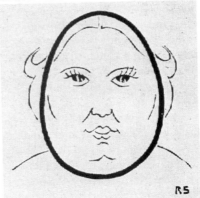

71

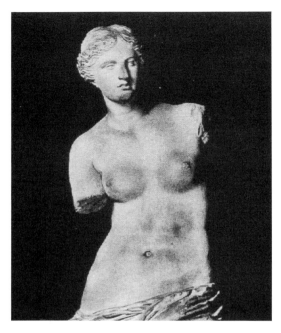

Venus of Milo (Louvre Museum, photo Bulloz)

swells towards the right, and projects below the upper lip in a sensual pout. The round full chin does not project, and has a dimple at its centre.

The delicately whorled ears are astonishingly small, but the lobes are fleshy.

The hair, black or dark chestnut, is fine, supple and abundant. It waves naturally and keeps its colour into old age.

The neck, perfectly round, merges into plump, sloping shoulders. The pectoral muscles of a man resemble those of a woman in shape and development. The woman looks her best in low-necked dresses. The whiteness of her throat, the roundness of her shoulders, the lively intelligent set of her back, all combine to give a strong impression of sensuality. The breasts, well-separated, low-slung and apple-shaped, seem to spring forward; they precede her like the throat of a pigeon. In old age her throat becomes fleshy and needs support.

Dimpled at shoulder and elbow, the arm ends in a slim, blue-veined wrist. The hands are

darken and go blue. The temples too are rounded and do not project.

The nose is straight and fairly big; broad at the base and rounded at the tip. It is plump, with mobile round open nostrils which may be fleshy and dilated.

Bright and moist, brown and lively, almost flush with the head, the almond-shaped eyes have dilated pupils. These are framed by round eyelids which project and are criss-crossed by a network of delicate blood-vessels. The long silky eyelashes curl backwards; the eyebrows, wide and well-defined, are some distance from the eyes, leaving a smooth uncovered space above the nose. The gaze of the Venusian is always soft and pleasant, but it can be winning and caressing, as voluptuous as the eye of an Andalusian.

The small round mouth, its cleft a wave which turns up at each end, is gently closed. The lips are plump, smooth and red. The teeth are small and close-fitting, their whiteness contrasting with the coral gums. In women the following is often seen: the lower lip, cleft in the middle,

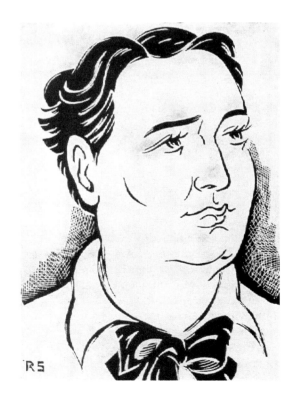

plump and dimpled, the fingers usually short, with spindle-shaped tips. The nails are generally curved and almond-shaped, the thumb is short. The skin is soft and white.

The loins are curved, the hips large and wide, the buttocks rounded. Musculature is not evident in the lower limbs. The thighs are large, long and rounded; the knees, with no knee-caps visible, bend slightly inwards, and the calves taper towards the small ankles; the feet are short and plump.

Kinetic

Inertia is the essential quality in the posture of a Venusian subject. The men have an effeminate appearance and manner; they enjoy mimicking, coquettish and provocative behaviour.

The gait is easy, supple and graceful. The Venusian walks with dancing steps. A woman proceeds with tranquil self-confidence inspired by the consciousness of her charm (but not of her social rank, as does the Jupiterian lady). Her undulant, rhythmical gait is recognisable at a distance.

Gestures are always graceful, charming and unhurried, sometimes marked by a touch of wantonness. A woman will throw her head back and look you in the face with a sweetness that naturally invites sympathy. Even during an argument she smiles with her eyes, for her thoughts are never grim or aggressive.

Venusian subjects dance well and easily, with shapely legs and elegant mobile ankles. They are also usually good singers. Their voices are sweet, tender and moderately pitched, with a pleasing seductive tone that captures the ear.

FUNCTIONS OF THE TYPE

Mind

Curiosity and a good memory are the outstanding mental faculties of Venusians; but this statement needs expanding. The curiosity which animates them is not scientific enquiry. Their minds are not fired by the desire for knowledge. They simply want to see new things, countries hitherto unknown to them, people whom they

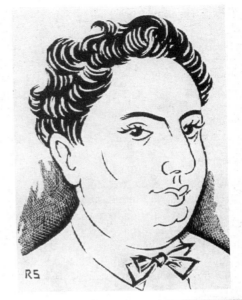

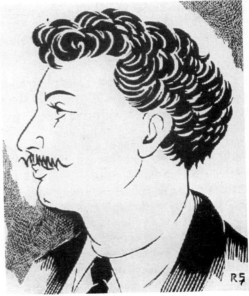

have not met before. Their curiosity is quite superficial. Nevertheless, they are always enchanted by beauty of form. Very sociable, and with an amiable manner, they love the world and its pleasures; parties have a great attraction for them. They like unusual and striking clothes, ornaments of all kinds, jewellery and pretty things, luxury in general;

73

although too often they prefer glitter to solid value.

Their intelligence, lively enough, is more brilliant than reliable; they include many talented people but few geniuses. It is in the field of the arts, especially music and the theatre, that they can become known and sometimes famous.

Their memory is well-behaved: they learn with ease, and forget as easily. In fact their memory will allow them to undertake major studies – if they want to. But after making a great effort, in order to please a parent or win a prize, they relapse again into their habitual inertia. Serious lectures bore them, and they find manual work exhausting. They detest solitude, and their imagination, purely sentimental in content, becomes overcast with gloom during a period of isolation, however short. Finally, they cling tenaciously to life and become very anxious when ill, because of their intense fear of death.

Character

Venusians have a horror of combat, hardship, fatigue and trouble. Very trusting, and easily deceived, they long for peace and quiet.

They are remarkably lucky people. Fortune seems to shower gifts upon them, and their success is often much greater than they deserve. Lighthearted, teasing, optimistic, with no worry for the future, they see everything in a rosy light. But their enthusiasm for pleasure and luxury can lead to egotism.

Expansive, demonstrative and sociable, they are naturally lovable and easy-going. They extend a ready welcome and are humane, affectionate and merciful. These natural tendencies are expressed in many ways: they laugh and weep easily; generous, even prodigal, they thoughtlessly promise more than they can ever fulfil, but will readily give of what they have, with pleasure, and without counting the cost.

They are frank and faithful friends, but inconstant lovers. They are gifted with charm and tenderness. The tall, dark, handsome Venusian seducer is also a clever actor. A good

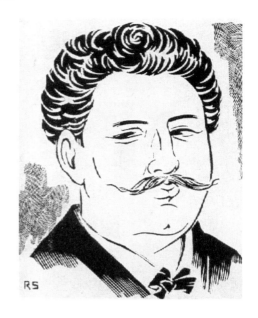

talker and an egotist, he knows how to play on the feelings of his victims. He pleases women and trusts to luck. La Bruyère was no doubt thinking of the Venusian type when he wrote, 'Women accuse men of being fickle, and the men reply that the women are shallow.' Venusians appear to be at once pious and worldly.

THE VENUSIAN WOMAN

Love is the great motivating force of the Venusian woman. You must not ask from her the profound sentiment of the Saturnian, nor the lyrical mysticism of Luna, nor the heroism of Mars, nor the cleverness of Mercury. She loves, and she lavishes her never-ending tenderness, finding all her happiness in giving to those around her. She loves, and her exquisite sensitivity supplies the rest. She is the ideal woman whom every man wants to marry for this one charming quality: she identifies with the one she loves and will give him all the joy he asks for.

There are no Venusians in convents, and none remain virgins. The Venusian girl, if pure and chaste, will hope to marry before having a

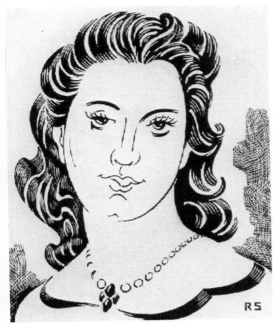

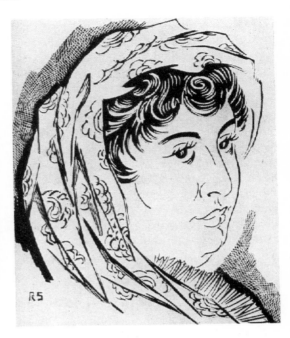

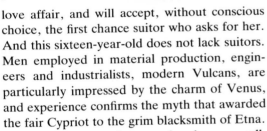

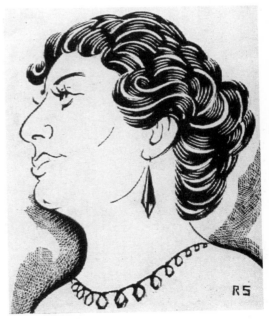

love affair, and will accept, without conscious choice, the first chance suitor who asks for her. And this sixteen-year-old does not lack suitors. Men employed in material production, engineers and industrialists, modern Vulcans, are particularly impressed by the charm of Venus, and experience confirms the myth that awarded the fair Cypriot to the grim blacksmith of Etna.

In contrast to Luna, who has a well-developed and exacting imagination, and to the Jupiterian lady who is preoccupied with social and worldly vanities, Venus seeks for nothing but the realisation of intimate joy. She wants to be loved sanely and peacefully, and will be a good wife as long as she is not burdened with one or both of two impossible conditions – abstinence and indifference. Venus must never be neglected, either morally or sensually. Her predilections are for flowers, perfumes and jewels. She enjoys exciting food, especially champagne. She likes to give intimate little parties, and her talent for pleasing people is shown by the way she prepares a surprise gift for each guest.

A sympathetic person who asks no more from life than reciprocated love, she incarnates joy for tender souls. Beautiful and gentle, she brings peace and smiles to the home. Luna may be dedicated to dreamers with complex desires; Apollo to intellectuals dominated by ideas; Jupiter to the ambitious, and Mercury to practical people. But loving hearts belong to the good Venus; not the adventuress who fills mythology with her amours, but the ideal woman who devotes herself to one man, her home and her children.

Venus (or Aphrodite – born from the foam of the sea) is one of the most celebrated deities of antiquity; it is she who presides over the pleasures of love. Mythology tells us that she wore a girdle which enclosed her graces and attractions: the engaging smile, the soft voice, the most persuasive sigh, the expressive silence and the eloquent eyes. These are the chief qualities of Venusians, which lend so much charm to their company.

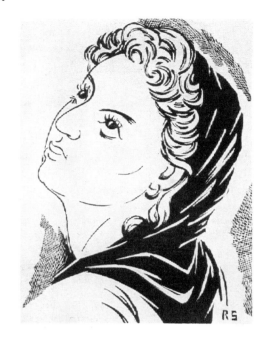

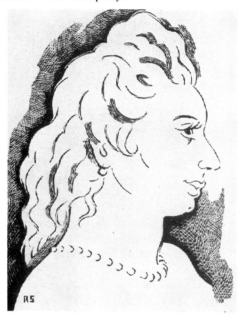

DISEASES AND REMEDIES OF VENUSIANS

Before studying the diseases and remedies of Venusians, one should be aware of how the type may be modified according to the constitution – Carbonic, Phosphoric or Fluoric.

Carbonic Constitution

Remember that one of the chief characteristics of the Venusian is indolence. The Carbonic

Venusian is gifted with extraordinarily powerful inertia. Nothing troubles or moves him. He lives his own small life: small, because he has no great ambitions; restricted, because he has a horror of effort; nor does he react to comments or expressions of disapproval. The natural resistance due to his Carbonic constitution allows him to bear philosophically any annoyance he may experience, whilst his hatred of conflict reinforces his egotistical desire to avoid all complications.

Phosphoric Constitution

The Phosphoric Venusian is far from being passive or inert. He can enthuse over an ideal, be it artistic or social, though he might not pursue it to completion if this demanded constant effort; and he will certainly take the trouble to use his natural qualities of curiosity and memory. He is a seeker, artistic or literary rather than scientific, an excellent historian or a gifted writer. Very sociable and persuasive, he can be trusted to shine in his chosen circles. Sensitive and sensual, he is always seeking new experiences, and whilst he avoids possessive women, pursues his conquests without thinking of the ravages that his superficial passion could create around him.

Fluoric Constitution

The Fluoric Venusian also seeks to use his gifts for ends which are not always justifiable. In political life his memory, which is faultless, allows him to recall annoying little incidents which have occurred in the lives of his colleagues. He knows how to use them to good purpose; thus he will triumph, in spite of his natural laziness, not through the authority of his personality but by his power to instil fear.

In daily life the Fluoric Venusian is a twister who seeks to draw profit from the efforts and failings of his contemporaries. Fortune smiles on him and he is successful.

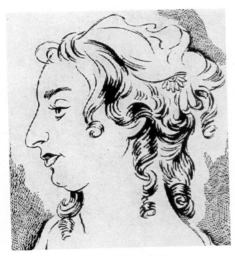

After Sir Peter Lely

TRANSMUTATIONS OF THE VENUSIAN

Morbid Predispositions

Physical Disorders

The well-known passivity of Venusians, coupled with their incorrigible laziness, ensures that they lead an unhealthy life. Frequent parties lead to excess, since though they may not be really greedy, they do enjoy good living and frothy sparkling wines. Champagne is their favourite drink. As a result they often suffer from stomach troubles and gout.

Furthermore, their sexual desires are frequent and powerful. They exhaust themselves and recover slowly. Physical exercise has no place in their lives and they are not given to sport. Finally they are subject to venereal disease, for Venusians, complex beings who are both sensual and lascivious, are not content just to satisfy their appetites, but multiply the occasions for doing so with consequences which may prove disastrous. The Venusian woman suffers from genital disorders which range from simple ovarian congestion to chronic metritis. Her periods are troublesome, usually too long and too abundant, and her labours are painful. In old age the Venusian becomes fat, her neck thickens, her cheeks fill out, her waist expands, walking becomes a torture, and cellulite makes its appearance and develops rapidly. If, when approaching the age of forty, she can resign herself to adopting the airs and graces of an older woman, Venus acquires a new talent – she knows how to age gracefully.

Psychological Disorders

The habitual inertia of Venusians leads to indolence. If they do not try to counteract this, if they give way to their baser instincts, they become lazy and flabby. They indulge in the lowest forms of sexuality without restraint, and will sacrifice everything to satisfy their insatiable lust. We know a young girl of nineteen who had run away from home on numerous occasions. Each time she ended up in an asylum. This poor wretch, who had a very well-balanced sister, was of Fluoric constitution and mentally retarded into the bargain. She was the despair of her mother who, having been widowed early in life, had to work all day and was thus unable to exercise proper supervision over the activities of her child.

The Venusian woman who lacks restraint and modesty is indeed a 'femme fatale'. She does not do evil for its own sake but for the profit she can gain from it. Her overriding egoism does not hesitate to sacrifice her lover to an unworthy

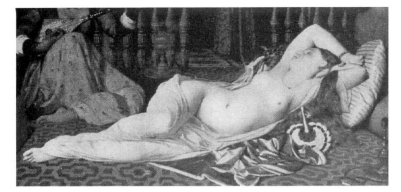

J.-D. Ingres
The Odalisque as a Slave,
fragment (Pereira Collection,
photo Bulloz)

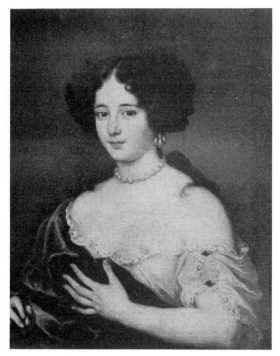

Marie Mancini as a Young Woman (Berlin,
photo Bulloz)

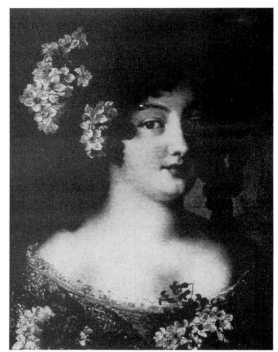

Pierre Mignard, *Marie Mancini*, fragment
(Kraemer collection, photo Bulloz)

fantasy. Courtesan by vocation, she knows how to awaken the senses, and to identify herself with them by consummate art. She appeals to the earthy instinct latent in every man, ensnaring him by clever and lascivious manipulation. She can be simultaneously loved to the point of suicide and despised to the point of murder.

Such are the moral maladies of the Venusian: vulgarity and sensuality, coquetry and rashness, together with a terrifying egoism which sacrifices everything to the satisfaction of the appetite.

Modifications of the Type

It comes as no surprise that in the Venusian, usually so good to look at, changes in appearance will alert the observer to a deviation from the normal type to one bearing unpleasant or wicked tendencies, such as would merit the 'inauspicious' description given by the ancient astrologers. In these cases the forehead becomes low and flat; the thick eyebrows meet, and the round, bright eyes emit a look of impudent desire. The nose turns up, the mouth widens and the coarse lips project. The tongue appears between the lips as if to caress them.

The gait, no longer harmonious and rhythmical, is marked by a provocative swing of the hips, revealing an abnormal development of the individual's posterior. You will easily recognise the skimming walk of these Venusian men and women and understand the reason for it. It is the gait of pederasts and prostitutes.

Whilst the normal Venusian woman is personally fastidious, as soon as she lets herself go with the rabble, be it ever so slightly, she becomes dirty and untidy. The delicate features coarsen, the heavy arm merges into a thick fist. The breasts hang down, flabby and voluminous. The waist expands and changes shape: a large belly in front and full buttocks behind; the short thighs end in knock-knees. The downfall is complete.

TREATMENT

Three basic remedies keep recurring in the treatment of Venusians: Calcarea Carbonica, Graphites and Thuja.

Calcarea Carbonica

Weakness, slowness and apathy are the dominant characteristics of the Calcarea Carbonica subject. Adolescents needing this remedy are not capable of vigorous exercise and detest sports, which they cannot easily practise because of their feeble muscles. They are subject to frequent colds and spend the winter coughing and blowing their noses. Slow and apathetic, as much from character as from the

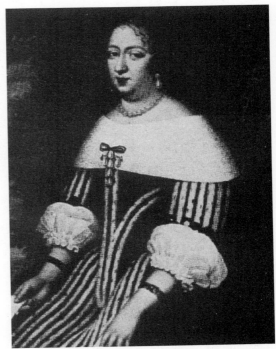

Nocret père, *Anne of Austria*, fragment (Versailles Museum, photo Nomis)

obesity which rapidly overtakes them, they only enjoy life if it is quiet, consisting of intellectual pursuits and daydreams. Good scholars and anaemic young girls often benefit from this remedy.

You will find the same characteristics in the adult, and especially in those young women who are sweet and sensitive, soft and indolent, and often acutely embarrassed by the flushes which rise to their faces after meals or in cold air. Periods are another source of distress to them – too frequent and too abundant, so that the sufferer is perpetually exhausted, but never ill enough to claim the sympathy of those around her.

When Calcarea Carbonica is closely studied in relation to the Venusian, two main groups of symptoms will be found: psychological troubles and menstrual disorders.

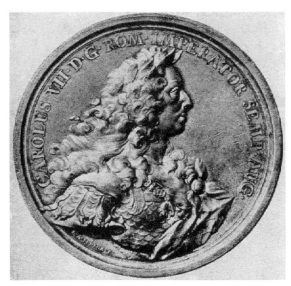

Charles VII, Emperor of Austria

Psychological Troubles

This subject has no memory, can hardly give his attention to anything, and is full of apprehension. The explanation is that he is apathetic, physically, intellectually and emotionally. He is lazy and slow-moving. Any form of activity seems impossible to him. He also has attacks of weakness which are not regular but may come on at any time, for instance when going upstairs, walking, or on making the slightest movement.

His apathy is not only physical but mental as well. He works slowly. He is full of good intentions but finds it difficult to study, for he cannot always remember what he has learned.

He also has trouble in keeping his attention fixed on anything. It is not that his mind wanders off to other subjects (like the patient who needs Calcarea Fluorica) – he simply cannot give his attention to the matter in hand. Not only this, mental work itself tires him out. There are young men of fourteen, fifteen or sixteen who ask for nothing better from life than to study. They understand well and would like to do well, but they cannot retain what they seek to learn and their work is unproductive. When they come as patients the family will tell you,

'When he makes a big mental effort, large drops of perspiration appear on his forehead.' That is an important symptom of Calcarea Carbonica: 'Hot head, and sweating from intellectual work'.

They also sometimes complain of headaches. Students may suffer from very severe headaches which diminish or disappear during a meal; this is the Anacardium headache. But note the difference between Anacardium and Calcarea Carbonica: the Anacardium patient has lost his memory, which used to be excellent; whereas the Calcarea Carbonica patient never had a memory at all. Anacardium cannot study because he immediately gets a headache, but Calcarea Carbonica does not get a headache at once. He makes a tremendous effort – this causes such congestion that he, who is usually chilly, perspires freely from his forehead and the next moment finds that he is suffering from pain in the head. Calcarea Carbonica is forgetful and cannot apply himself. He cannot count, or multiply, or solve a little problem, since he cannot retain the images of the figures which he has just seen.

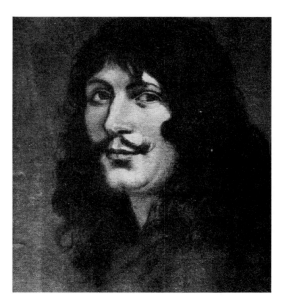

Le Guerchin, Self-portrait, (Chantilly, Condé Museum, photo Braun)

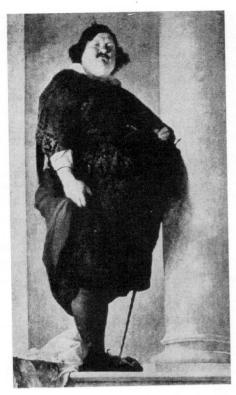

Velasquez, *Alexandro del Borro* (Berlin, photo Giraudon)

Another important characteristic is apprehension. What kind of apprehension? This subject certainly fears the future. He is anxious. He is afraid of catching illnesses. Or else he is afraid that something disastrous will happen to his business. In these moments of anxiety, of anguish for the future, he has palpitations.

The explanation for this apprehension is that it denotes a true mental weakness, which prevents him from studying. He is aware of this flaw that brings all his intellectual efforts to nothing, and is afraid that others will see it and recognise his incapacity.

He is also afraid of losing his reason, and again fears that others will notice it. Here we are reminded of another remedy: Actaea Racemosa. This woman patient is also afraid of going mad, especially at the change of life. She has terrible headaches, and pain in the ovaries.

This tendency of Calcarea Carbonica to believe that those around him will think him insane is explained by the fact that he does show a series of mental aberrations. He sometimes has bizarre impulses, as in the following example. A child walks quietly along the edge of the pavement, then suddenly starts to run, no one knows why, and then as suddenly stops, again without anyone knowing why. Or else there is the young man who runs upstairs very quickly, as if in terror. Then there is the patient who constantly repeats the same movement, or who entertains himself for a whole day making pigs out of breadcrumbs, or rolling up little balls of paper, or who will sit for hours in a corner nursing a doll or a piece of velvet. He is always busy with some small, constantly repeated manual task. These signs are also met with in manic depressives.

The Calcarea Carbonica patient also suffers from hallucinations. They are usually visual hallucinations in full waking consciousness. He sees people walking beside him, and thinks that someone is trying to pass him in the street. (Petroleum also has this feeling of someone beside him.)

The Calcarea Carbonica subject is compelled to think of ridiculous things which torment him and prevent him from working. Thus he will dwell on animals and insects, or on assassins and adventure stories he may have read. Once he has become obsessed with these thoughts he has difficulty in escaping from them.

To sum up, Calcarea Carbonica is weak. He cannot fix his attention, and his apathy and slowness prevent him from working. He is anxiously aware of this cerebral disturbance and very apprehensive that others will notice it too.

Menstrual Disorders

The Calcarea Carbonica patient's periods are always early, prolonged and heavy, accompanied by a feeling of localised coldness in the legs and feet that persists even when she is in bed. Silicea suffers similarly from feelings of coldness during the periods. But whereas in Calcarea Carbonica the sensation is localised in

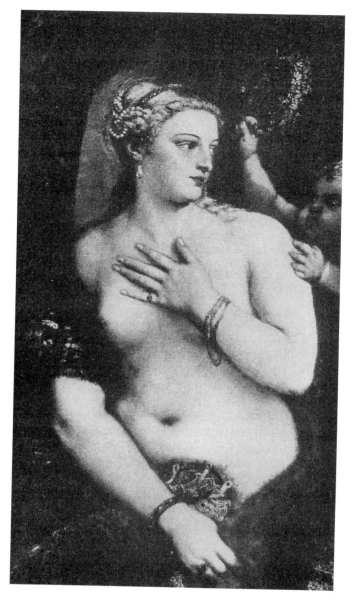

Titian
The Adornment of Venus, fragment
(St Petersburg, Hermitage Museum,
photo Giraudon)

the extremities, in Silicea it is general. The patient is always freezing during her period, even in summer.

Which are the remedies to be compared with Calcarea Carbonica? Calcarea Phosphorica naturally comes first to mind. The period is early in Calcarea Phosphorica, and the blood is bright red, sometimes blackish. The other well-known symptoms of Calcarea Phosphorica should be sought for: aggravation of troubles when thinking of them, desire for smoked and salt meat, a gurgling distended belly, frequent diarrhoea, leucorrhoea like white of egg.

Nux Vomica also has early periods, which last for a long time, but they are usually irregular, and the blood is black instead of bright red.

82

Rhus Toxicodendron has early prolonged periods which are associated with attacks of genital herpes. Rhus Tox. also sometimes has sharp pains at the top of the vagina at the beginning of a period.

Platina has heavy periods that appear as black clots, accompanied by spasms and a sensation of pressure from below. Platina has vaginal hypersensitivity, which may make intercourse impossible, associated with sexual hyperexcitability. It should also be remembered that Platina sees objects as much smaller than they really are. She is usually a haughty person who knows infinitely better than any doctor the treatment and way of life she should follow.

Secale (ergot, a parasite of rye) corresponds to heavy irregular periods with black blood, and followed by a watery discharge which lasts for a

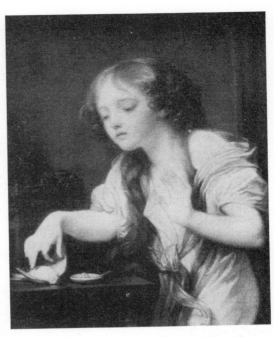

Greuze, *The Dead Bird* (Louvre Museum, photo Bulloz)

long time, sometimes even until the beginning of the next period. Secale patients are emaciated. They are always cold, but in spite of feeling cold, present a total intolerance to heat. They are much worse for being covered up, and need to have the windows open.

Sepia should be mentioned here. This is surprising, as Sepia's periods are nearly always late, with a sensation of weight in the pelvis. Nevertheless, in some cases Sepia may usefully be given. For instance, if a patient shows all the symptoms of Sepia except that her periods are early, this should not be taken for a contradictory symptom, since in some cases the periods are heavy and early. But in Sepia these heavy, early periods will be associated with another clinically important symptom – prolapse of the uterus. This is a major indication for Sepia, and it is a symptom which is not only subjective (a feeling of weight in the pelvis), but also clinical, in that you are in fact dealing with a uterus which is large, congested and prolapsed. Note also the milky leucorrhoea charac-

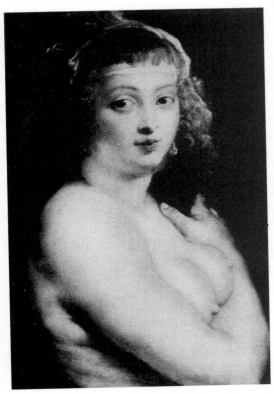

Rubens, *Hélène Fourment*, fragment (Vienna, photo Viollet)

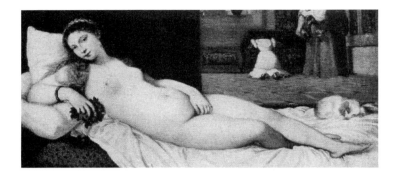

Titian
The Venus of Urbino,
fragment (Florence, Uffizzi
Museum, photo Bulloz)

teristic of Sepia, which appears before, rather than after, the period.

Ferrum Metallicum also has early periods, found in women who are very frail and anaemic. They have pale faces which may suddenly become red – pallor alternates with flushing. The colour of the menstrual blood is not bright red, as in Calcarea Carbonica or Nux Vomica, but pale. The periods of Ferrum have the distinctive quality that they are intermittent – they stop, and start again two days later. Intermittence also recalls Pulsatilla, and sometimes it may be difficult to choose between Ferrum and Pulsatilla, even though the objective and functional symptoms are quite different. In Ferrum the periods are heaviest at night, whereas in Pulsatilla they are heavier by day and cease almost completely during rest at night.

Belladonna has abundant, heavy periods. The blood is bright red and shows another characteristic peculiar to Belladonna – it is hot. The patient feels that a hot liquid is flowing from her vagina in large quantities. She will show the other symptoms of Belladonna too, such as flushes of heat, beating of the carotid arteries, etc.

Millefolium also has very heavy periods. This is a remedy for any haemorrhage (vaginal, uterine, pulmonary). Very painful vaginal varices which become worse during pregnancy are one local symptom. Note that the headache of Millefolium is relieved by epistaxis, in contrast to the Borax headache, which comes on after epistaxis.

Ipecacuanha also has early heavy periods with bright red blood. Thus Ipecacuanha presents exactly the same symptoms as Belladonna or Calcarea Carbonica. But Ipecacuanha has the additional characteristic symptom of nausea and even vomiting with a clean red tongue.

Sabina is a remedy for menorrhagia and metrorrhagia with bright blood. It gives good results where there are bleeding fibroids. The patient experiences a painful sensation in the vagina, from below upwards, as if something was pressing into it. This is different from the symptom of Sepia, who feels a sensation of pressure from above downwards. The Sepia patient also has a pain from the sacrum to the pubis, as if she was transfixed from back to front. This pain of transfixion from back to front can be contrasted with the pains which go from left to right or from right to left, as found in Trillium Pendulum. It is as if the hips were being pulled apart, so much so that the patient has to bandage them. Trillium Pendulum also has metrorrhagia, and where there are fibroids, large clots of bright red blood. Bright red blood is thus found in Belladonna, Millefolium, Ipecacuanha, Sabina and Trillium Pendulum. The main objective characteristics of these five remedies are the same. But less important symptoms, as indicated above, often allow them to be differentiated.

Thlaspi Bursa Pastoris also has menorrhagia and metrorrhagia; the periods are heavy and painless with large clots of black blood. These periods last for from ten to fifteen days, and the haemorrhage is more abundant in every alternate period. The exhausted patient barely has time to recover from one bleeding before the next one starts.

Such are the principal remedies indicated in the Venusian woman.

Graphites

Venusians gain weight with age. A double chin appears, the belly bulges, cellulite develops, and the patient becomes progressively more obese. Lassitude and indolence are more marked, they take no exercise and remain seated or lying down, renouncing all further physical or intellectual activity. They certainly continue to live, but in a vegetative way, indifferent to all that goes on around them, anxious only about themselves and their well-being, sad and restless.

Now think of the characteristics of Graphites: an apathetic, fat, chilly constipated person; her periods are late, scanty and short, with constantly oozing leucorrhoea; sticky ulcers have yellowish discharge, viscous and thick like honey; eczema oozes from many areas – behind the ears, on the scalp, the eyelashes, the lips, the chin, the flexures of the limbs, the genitalia, and between the fingers and toes. The totality of these morbid symptoms is unmistakeably an exaggeration of the signs of Calcarea Carbonica. These two remedies seem to succeed one another in the life of a patient. Calcarea Carbonica is a great remedy of childhood and adolescence; in adult life its therapeutic effect recedes, and in old age it may even be harmful. Graphites in its total symptom picture is predominantly a remedy for mature people, and its indications are seen most often in the patient whose organism has achieved a stable balance; through cutaneous elimination it counteracts the effects of intestinal blockage and the cessation of periods. It has been said that Graphites is the Pulsatilla of the menopause. Both are incontestably useful remedies for regulation and drainage.

It is a curious fact that whilst the Calcarea Carbonica patient hates the cold, Pulsatilla is made worse by heat. If the two remedies are

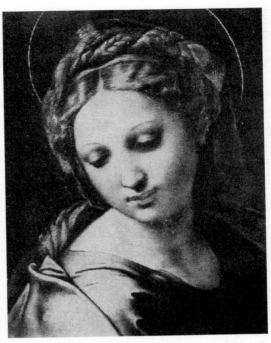

Raphael, *The Virgin*, detail from the Holy Family called 'The Pearl' (Madrid, Prado Museum, photo Anderson)

carefully compared, a similarity with inverse modalities will be found. Localisation to a mucous surface in a Calcarea Carbonica subject often requires the use of Pulsatilla.

Calcarea Carbonica, Pulsatilla and Graphites – a felicitous sequence of complementary remedies, demonstrate the changes that occur with time, especially in the Venusian.

Genital complaints are often found in Venusians. They include chronic urethritis, which can turn a man into a urinary invalid, and utero-ovarian infection, which has lasting debilitating effects on a woman. These conditions require the use of a number of remedies which cannot all be studied here. Hydrastis, Helonias, Natrum Sulphuricum and Medorrhinum are the principal agents to which we most often have recourse. But there is one remedy which is perfectly adapted to the morbid transformation which takes place in Venusians of both sexes – Thuja.

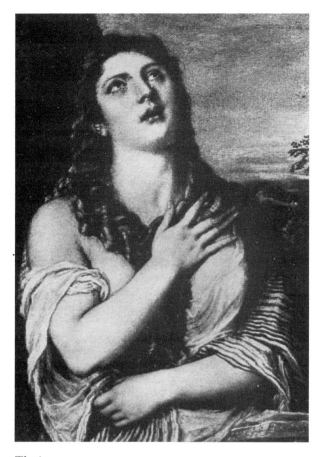

Titian
Mary Magdalene, fragment
(St Petersburg, Hermitage
Museum, photo Giraudon)

Thuja

This is the remedy for corpulent people whose fat is mostly on the thighs and buttocks and who have developed a generalised cellullite. The face is oily and shining, the alae nasi carry numerous varicosities, the nasolabial fold is accentuated. The hair is greasy and full of dandruff, the veins start out on the limbs, the hands are cold and sticky. But this is not only a physical transformation – there is also a real psychological change. The Venusian who has previously lived as he pleased, carefree and lazy, becomes preoccupied, anxious and restless. This tendency becomes stronger and stronger, turning into an obsession with futile and ridiculous things. Fixed ideas take root in his mind, changing every two or three days according to the cause which has triggered them – loss of a treasured object, a broken vase, a word heard and wrongly interpreted . . .

The idea of sex dominates the Venusian and rapidly becomes an obsession if unsatisfied. Staphysagria is the remedy here. Similarly, Lachesis will prove very useful when unreasoning jealousy disrupts conjugal relations and threatens to shatter the equilibrium of a family. This subject is excessively hypersensitive. He cannot sleep, and will wake regularly at 4 a.m.

Later, slowly but progressively, a profound modification of his whole being takes place, a cancerous state which culminates in the appearance of a tumour. Morphologists have maintained that the round, hunch-backed individual was predisposed to cancer. Venusians, who are rounded people, are indeed more inclined than others to cancerous disease, to which they are naturally susceptible because of the impregnation of the organism as a result of genital disease.

Life Style

It is difficult to establish healthy living in such an indolent, apathetic person. However, certain rules should be followed if the Venusian man or woman is to be properly balanced.

Regular exercise can be prescribed, to replace sexual stimulation by healthy fatigue, but it will soon be given up. The physician would do better to try and counteract artificial stimulants, and should warn against the abuse of strong pervasive perfumes which tend to increase sexual desire, and to which Venusians are particularly partial. It makes no sense to seek, by stimuli which rapidly become harmful, to increase activities which are already temperamentally well developed.

In conclusion it must be admitted that a healthy way of life, however necessary, will be difficult for the Venusian subject to observe in practice. Happily, the homoeopathic doctor possesses important remedies for preventing pathological developments which would otherwise end fatally. These include Calcarea Carbonica and Graphites, although the great basic remedy for Venusians will always be Thuja, whose remedial action prevents the development of tumours.

REMEDIES OF THE VENUSIAN

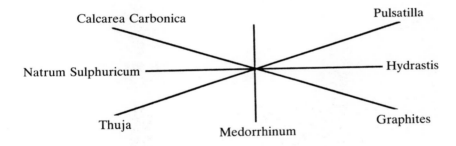

Calcarea Carbonica   Pulsatilla

Natrum Sulphuricum   Hydrastis

Thuja   Medorrhinum   Graphites

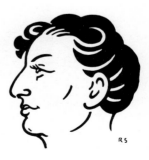

8

Jupiter

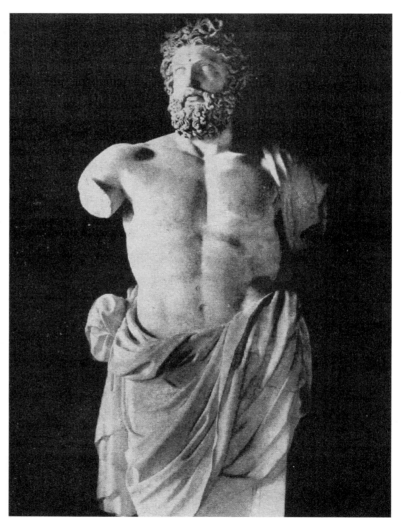

Bust of Jupiter, known as *Jupiter of Versailles*
(Paris, Louvre Museum, photo Viollet)

Jupiter is Master of the Gods, enthroned on the cloudy peak of Mount Olympus, from which the earth is suspended by golden chains. His frown causes Olympus to tremble. Majestic, hirsute and bearded, he mediates between heaven and earth, contemplating divine unity in the multiplicity of things under his control. He possesses beauty without being possessed by it; working with society as man works with matter, he manages the external world in the same way that the intellectual manages his internal world. Thus Jupiter dethrones Saturn.

Jupiter is the moving spirit in a body at rest, the calm leader who gets things done. Like Louis XIV, or the President of some Trust, sitting at his desk while he mobilises a world of men and things. Louis XIV, Goethe, Leonardo da Vinci, Prud'homme – all were Jupiterians.

DOMINANT CHARACTERISTICS

Medium height.
Majestic, Olympian demeanour.
Heavy, solemn gait.
Cheerful, bold and jovial. Optimistic, practical, dominating.

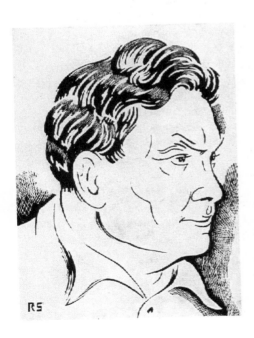

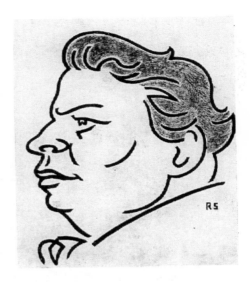

DESCRIPTION

Medium height (1.65–1.75m in a man). Majestic, imposing attitude. Solemn, heavy gait with corresponding gestures, alternating from right to left and vice versa. His face is the shape of an acorn. High wide forehead. Square skull, with vertex slightly domed. Small nose, aquiline or straight. Flaring nostrils. Fairly large mouth. Strong, rounded firm lips. Rounded chin, which may recede somewhat. Heavy ears with flat lobes. Soft brown curly hair. Light brown eyebrows which dive towards the nose. Wide-open grey eyes. Fresh rosy complexion. High strong chest. Strong muscular arms. Square fleshy hands. Heavy legs. Small fat feet.

MORPHOLOGY

Static

Of medium build and well proportioned, if sometimes somewhat corpulent, the Jupiterian stands out on account of his dignity. Whatever his social background, his appearance is not only correct but has a certain nobility that commands respect.

Seen from the front, his wide, fleshy face appears to be square, but the total shape of his head can be compared to that of an acorn. His

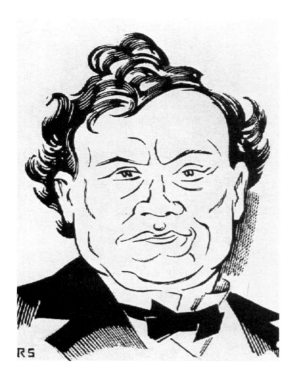

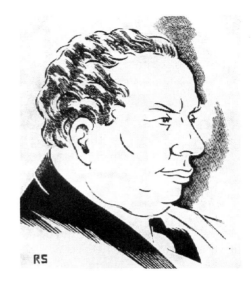

skull is well-proportioned and lightly domed; high in the sub-occipital region, and more brachycephalic than dolichocephalic. His forehead is handsome, well-proportioned as to height and width. It describes a noble curve, with eminences on the right and left sides. His hair is brown or ruddy blond, supple, thick and wavy or curly. But the Jupiterian tends to premature hair loss, and the first bald patch is to be found on the top of his head.

The eyebrows are a fair distance above the eyes, well grown and gently arched. They are generally calm and serene, but frown slightly when Jupiter reprimands. The eyes are large, handsome, laughing and moist; wide open but not protruding; of a greyish colour, or sometimes dark blue; framed by thick eyelids. His gaze is straight and open, denoting firmness and benevolence, always with a hint of fun.

His elegantly-shaped nose is fairly short, and may be straight or aquiline, with thick, dilated hairy nostrils. A big chin completes this noble face, whose firm hairy cheeks cover powerful

jaws. If the chin is straight or projects forward slightly, the subject will have a forceful character; if it recedes, he may lack will-power. But the abiding characteristic of the Jupiterian face lies in its frank and open expression, radiating health and cheerfulness, and in its florid complexion, which may also burgeon with generally itchy eruptions.

His ears are quite heavy, with flat lobes. His neck is strong and powerful, but at the same time elegant and shapely. Marked with bluish veins, it surmounts a big hairy chest. In a woman the breasts are high and firm and very solid, covered with a fine, pinkish-white skin.

The shoulders are strong and hairy, the back massive and powerful; the supple, muscular arms are rather short. The hands are thick and solid; square palms terminate in square-tipped fingers, which are thick at the base and often long.

The hips are large; the relatively short legs are heavy and subject to varicosities. The calves are solid and muscular, the ankles massive, but the feet are small and fat.

Kinetic

The Jupiterian is typically a worthy man, imposing, sometimes solemn, Olympian but rarely arrogant, unless he has lost his usual good humour and been deformed by pride. His bearing commands respect, whilst the laughing, jovial expression of his face tempers to some extent the severity of his attitude. His gait is always ponderous. Jupiterians walk with their heads held high, unpretentiously, looking straight ahead or sometimes upwards.

Their gestures are direct and usually symmetrical. When speaking they often rub or clap their hands, as a sign of approbation or to show their joy. They have a real need for communication, and are constantly expressing it. Jupiterian children clap their hands and jump for joy when they are told good news. Their free, musical laughter is always accompanied by joyful gestures. But nothing will induce them to break the conventions, which they observe by a sort of instinct. Docile at lessons, attentive to criticism and anxious to avoid it, they give great satisfaction to their families. Another gesture typical of the successful and rather conceited Jupiterian is that of putting his hands in his braces, or in the sides of his waistcoat. Then whilst he is talking he adopts an aggressive attitude, or displays his vanity with satisfaction.

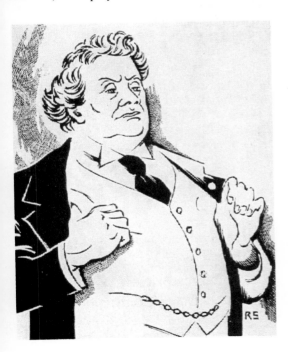

It is noteworthy that Jupiterians sweat easily, from the chest and the head, especially the forehead. Puberty is of early onset, and with age they acquire a good deal of weight and a double chin.

The Jupiterian voice is sonorous and harmonious. Warm and penetrating, it is admirably suited to orators. Its tonal quality is balanced and wide-ranging – grave or joyful, it is always easy to listen to.

The shape of a Jupiterian changes gradually with age. A tendency to overweight, indeed to obesity, is shown by men and women whose figures develop to their full extent.

THE JUPITERIAN FUNCTION

Mind

Practical intelligence is the dominant faculty of Jupiter. The mind is reflective and judicious, and gravity is tempered with benevolence. When they criticise it is with genuine authority and in a paternal manner. There is something in them which commands respect and dominates the souls of less discerning people. They deserve to command others, because they are in command of themselves.

Always reasonable, anxious to do the right thing and to be thought well of by their contemporaries, they reflect before speaking, taking a decision or giving advice. They are wise and prudent; often religious, they take pleasure in the ceremonies of the Church.

In the game of life the Jupiterian is a winner. He enjoys his work as well as the reward it brings, and delights in tackling problems. He often achieves his goal, and it is not rare to see Jupiter in the ascendant. If they are of modest birth or social status, Jupiterians will rise above it and come out of their obscurity, often by good luck as much as by merit alone. Fortune seems to smile upon them. In business undertakings they are often successful beyond their expectations. They have within themselves a ray of good fortune which leads to success in everything they do, and this seems to extend to all those under their protection, to whom they seem to be able to communicate a little of their own good luck.

Always good-humoured, they bring joy and prosperity to society. They speak wisely and at length, without having prepared a discourse;

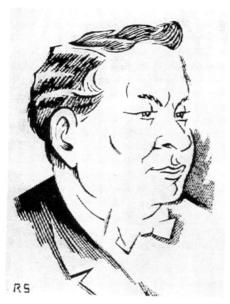

their words come from the heart, and their penetrating warmth encourages the timorous. Their natural seriousness does not prevent them from having a fund of funny stories to tell, calculated to make the audience laugh without blushing. They are great lovers of family life, cherishing their children and inclined to be over-indulgent with them. They enjoy reunions, where they are always given the place of honour, and meetings and assemblies, where they occupy the front seats. Brilliant, often superficial, able to assimilate facts quickly, they are tough and open-minded, sometimes reckless but always practical. Their aptitude is for moral and political sciences, jurisprudence and the administration of public affairs. A great many of them choose the church as their profession and rise to the highest positions within it.

Character

Essentially an optimist, the Jupiterian always hopes and never despairs. Hope is the faithful companion of his nature. He has a serene mind, full of confidence and usually occupied with pleasant thoughts.

His instinct for self-preservation is well-developed, which enables him to keep strict

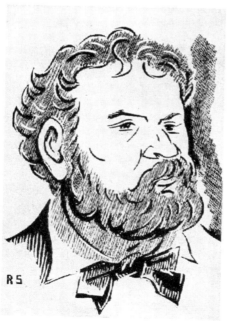

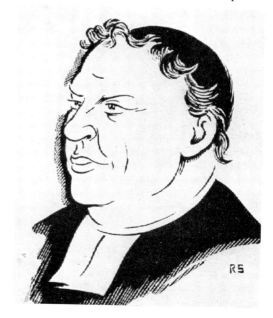

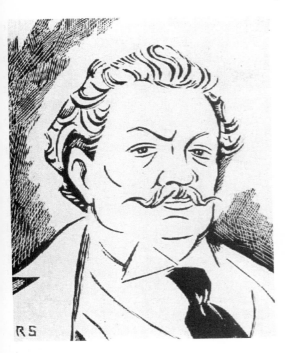

control over his voluptuous and greedy instincts. He clings to life and knows how to enjoy it, indeed he has difficulty in believing that he will ever have to die, so strongly does he reject the idea of death.

Jupiterians are natural Epicureans. Although subject to numerous temptations, they take their pleasures moderately and with reserve. They enjoy good meals in the company of merry companions and appreciate fine wines and good cooking; but they are cautious, and avoid even minor excesses. Although they love readily, and are loved in return, they do not want entanglements or worries. The Jupiter of mythology was suitably married to his own sister, but he did not disdain from seeking distraction amongst his subjects, such as Danae, Leda, Antiope and Semele.

They value kindness and conventional behaviour, and are easily upset if these are lacking; protocol must always be respected. They are good company; and affable, with children as well as with adults, and courteous towards women. They are also indulgent and forgive offences easily, in fact often do not remember them!

They have the instinct of property. If they desire riches it is not to hoard them but to use them for the common good. Money is for them a means to fulfil their vocation and create good conditions around themselves.

They are ambitious, primarily for a good reputation. Jealous of their authority, they will not allow it to be questioned. They are always under control, and watch their own reactions, using on themselves their keen and critical powers of observation. This is how they manage to repress the bouts of impatience to which they are subject.

According to their means, they like their surroundings to be impeccable, luxurious, or simply comfortable, preferring spacious rooms where light and air can penetrate freely. They surround themselves with fine statues and beautiful pictures; they have good taste in jewellery, and favour gentle perfumes which do not intoxicate. The colours they prefer are blue and purple. They especially value cleanliness and white linen; the order which rules their households is a reflection of the greater order to which their souls aspire. It goes without saying that their attire is never neglected, always simple, elegant and in good taste.

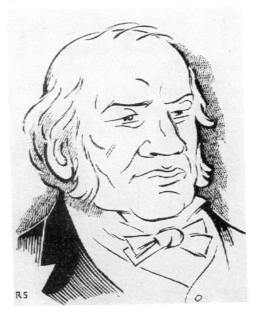

THE JUPITERIAN WOMAN

The best examples of Jupiterian women were to be found at the court of Louis XIV. The female Jupiterian of today will make a good wife for a senior civil servant or administrator, or indeed anyone in a high position, for she unites the qualities of resolution and elegance which are needed on all occasions. Her manner, correct for the great lady or ambassador's wife, would appear pretentious or over-formal in a middle-class setting, and ridiculously affected among working people. She is an accomplished woman of the world, and a perfect hostess.

Well-built without being too heavy, of medium size and correctly proportioned, the Jupiterian woman looks good and her usual manner is benevolent and protective. Her hair whitens easily but the face remains smooth and unlined for a long time. At fifty she is still attractive, and her tact, good manners and fastidiousness are retained into old age.

Her domestic virtues are very real, but her exterior life is played out in the world of audiences and functions. No other woman entertains so well and so graciously; her guests are always people of high degree, officials and celebrities. She likes to do things on a large

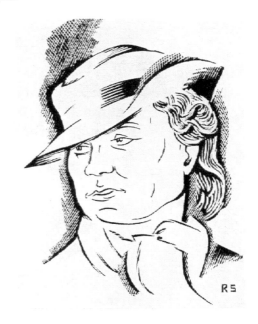

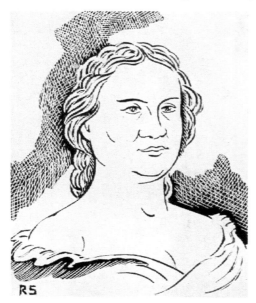

scale and may overspend her allowance, but she also supervises the office, verifies the bills, and is a good administrator. She keeps up with current fashion in matters of ceremony and decor, and favours a show of opulence. Cheerful and bold, the Jupiterian woman has great self-confidence. She does not know what it means to be timid, she believes in success, and will attempt the most foolhardy projects and get away with them. 'She is lucky,' they say. Yes, but this is the luck of fearless people who brave danger by brushing it out of the way, without a thought that someone or something might have to suffer for it.

Madam Carefree would be a good name for the common Jupiterian woman. She is at ease everywhere, rules everyone, dominates everything. 'Give her a foot and she will take a yard.' But she is such a good, warmhearted, spirited girl, so frank and energetic, that her despotism and anger are soon forgotten. With her the sun will surely shine after the storm! Gifted with worldly wisdom, she wilts in isolation. She needs to entertain and to visit people. Her imagination is not given to dreaming, for all her plans depend upon the mood of the social circle in which she moves.

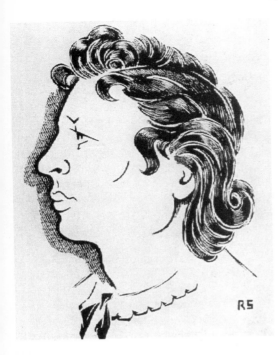

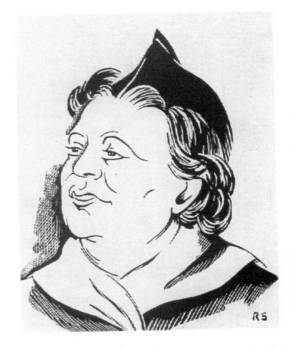

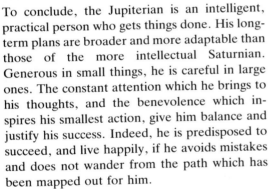

To conclude, the Jupiterian is an intelligent, practical person who gets things done. His long-term plans are broader and more adaptable than those of the more intellectual Saturnian. Generous in small things, he is careful in large ones. The constant attention which he brings to his thoughts, and the benevolence which inspires his smallest action, give him balance and justify his success. Indeed, he is predisposed to succeed, and live happily, if he avoids mistakes and does not wander from the path which has been mapped out for him.

DISEASES AND REMEDIES OF THE JUPITERIAN

Before beginning our study, it is necessary to understand the pattern which determines the constitution to which our Jupiterian belongs: Carbonic, Phosphoric or Fluoric.

Carbonic Constitution

The Carbonic Jupiterian is essentially reasonable, which makes sense when we recall the outstanding quality which governs all the actions of a Carbonic – he knows how to discipline and manage himself. The Jupiterian by his nature knows how to control his instincts and passions. The Carbonic Jupiterian chooses his company so as not to be tempted to the excesses to which he may be naturally prone. The habitual stolidity of the Carbonic is easily modified by the habitual cheerfulness of the Jupiterian. Anxious to do the right thing, he knows how to shoulder his responsibilities, always after lengthy consideration.

Phosphoric Constitution

The practical intelligence of a Jupiterian will compensate the bursts of enthusiasm which habitually animate the Phosphoric. For once, the Phosphoric appears as a realist. The artist, whatever his mode of expression – music, painting, sculpture or poetry – knows how to display his gifts to best advantage. His personality is likely to lead him to vanity, but the praise which he bestows upon himself (and generally deserves) will be so naive that he is immediately forgiven.

Fluoric Constitution

The Fluoric Jupiterian succeeds in everything he undertakes. Endowed with rapid assimilation, he judges promptly and acts quickly, but his love of money may lead him into practices which progressively affect his health. His vanity is inflated by the triumphs which he scores in all directions. Display and assertiveness soon become the guiding lines of his conduct. Instead of using his money to do good, he spends it on often ridiculous luxuries in order to dazzle his contemporaries, who soon make him the target of their jealousy.

TRANSMUTATIONS OF THE JUPITERIAN

On seeing a Jupiterian, everyone exclaims, 'What a fine man!' A Jupiterian woman similarly evokes the cry, 'What a lovely girl!' And indeed, Jupiter, with his gaiety, his good humour, his enjoyment of rich living and his easy pleasures, seems destined to enjoy life for a long time. Alas, this will not be the case unless he is sensible and can put a brake upon his natural tendencies.

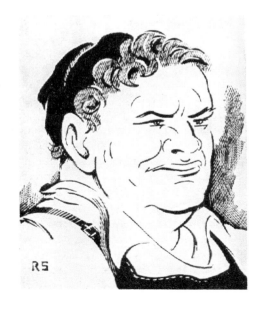

Morbid Predispositions

Physical Disorders

With age the Jupiterian puts on weight, gaining a large belly and a double chin. This excess of fat, which makes him heavier, is associated with a general accumulation of toxins. He becomes gouty and often diabetic. Like all sanguine people he is at risk of apoplexy and cardiac disorder. Do you suppose this worries him? In matters of health and strength he has no fears, neither for himself nor for others. He has been carved out of limestone and sand to live for a hundred years, and does not listen to the advice of his physician.

The Jupiterian becomes ill from living too well. He eats too much, of a diet that is rich and rare; he drinks too much strong alcoholic liquor. He does not get drunk, and rarely suffers from indigestion, but one fine day he will have a liver attack, or a sudden rise of blood pressure. To make matters worse, this patient is rarely in the habit of taking physical exercise. He much prefers to be a spectator.

The diseases which lie in wait for him are the rewards of his excesses: albuminuria, diabetes, gallstones, arrhythmia, arterial hypertension, apoplexy. Healthy crises of elimination occur, in the form of itching, rashes, gout, haemorrhoids or eczema, and their suppression by external treatment can lead to serious complications.

The Jupiterian woman, who looks very healthy but has an underlying low resistance, is predisposed to the same troubles. She has easy labours, but is prone to haemorrhages which recur at each menstrual period, or between them. This represents a healthy elimination of toxins, but she dreads it on account of the temporary weakness she experiences, and which is so foreign to her nature.

Psychological Disorders

The overriding malady of the Jupiterian is vanity. How could he escape it, a man who has risen from nowhere, and yet by the middle of his life occupies a commanding position in the community?

Happy to be alive, rejoicing in his triumphs, complacently aware of the position he has gained wihout having dared to hope for it, he treats his contemporaries ostentatiously but without scorn. With his watch-chain hanging over his bulging belly, and thumbs tucked into the seams of his waistcoat, he pontificates solemnly, unaware of the ridiculous figure he cuts. Louis XIV and Joseph Prud'homme express the Jupiterian formula: the one royal and grandiose, the other middle-class and a figure of fun.

An animal whose instincts are thwarted becomes vicious, whilst a man who does not discover how to use his faculties exemplifies disorder. Of course he is unhappy, because he has lost the way which had been traced for him, but he may also be wicked and dangerous. Similarly, the Jupiterian woman, by nature a leader in society and public life, becomes manipulative and perverse if destiny thwarts her claims. Her vanity will seek satisfaction in other directions. She will try to obtain the money she desires by dubious efforts of inheritance, such as conscientiously caring for an aged relative whose difficult behaviour she will tolerate, whilst at the same time longing for his or her death. When age and failure have condemned her to satisfy her need for superiority in a derisory manner, then her wickedness can equal that of the vindictive elderly Saturnine spinster.

Jupiterians who have lost control of their natural instincts become grossly sensual and greedy, and drink heavily. They talk loudly, seasoning their speech with jokes, odious puns and smutty stories, laughing uproariously at their own wit. Self-indulgent and shameless, they are the despair of their family. Their friends are mostly boon companions. Very ambitious, avid for money, clever, cunning, and especially lucky in business, they succeed where

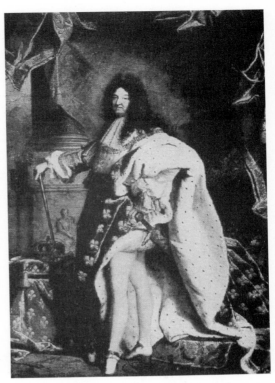

H. Rigaud, *Louis XIV* (Paris, Louvre Museum, photo Bulloz)

others fail. Boastful and cowardly, irreligious through false human respect, they fear death, and will call for a priest in their last moments.

Modifications of the Type

The moral transformation of a Jupiterian cannot take place without a profound modification of the type as described. The description itself does not change, but certain traits are accentuated, whilst others become less prominent or else disappear. The body is heavier, the expression haughty or off-hand. The protective attitude is still there, proud but more disdainful. The eyes are large and level with the face – in anger they appear to bulge outwards. The nose is shorter, the mouth big and sensual; the lips are thick, with the lower one projecting beyond the upper. The cheeks are very plump. The chin, square, fat and often double, is imperious,

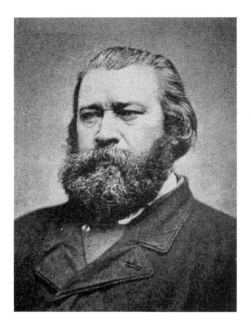

The Painter J.-F. Millet

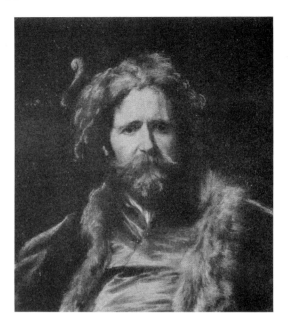

Van Dyck, *The Painter David Rickaert*, fragment
(Prado Museum, photo Anderson-Viollet)

even severe. The complexion becomes darker and may be blotchy. Bald from an early age, threatened by obesity which increases with their habitual way of life, Jupiterians still stand out amongst their contemporaries. Great eaters and great enjoyers, their main concern is to satisfy their appetites, which are certainly not delicate. Lacking in moral sense, they seek for honours and positions due to them. Rather than resign herself to a life without activity or glamour, the Jupiterian woman, a plotter rather than a heroine, will calmly commit atrocious crimes.

TREATMENT

Remedies of the Jupiterian

Against the moral malady of the Jupiterian, which is vanity, no remedy can be prescribed other than strong self-discipline. On the other hand, a physician can fight successfully against the bodily disorders which threaten the Jupiterian, unexpectedly shortening the life of someone who would otherwise appear to be a very resistant person indeed. Excess of all kinds

ends by causing a state of intoxication whose early manifestations are confusing.

Sulphur

The subject appears the picture of health, strong, robust, with a high colour, rosy lips and red ears. He is corpulent, cheery, optimistic, and does not look ill; nevertheless he tends to feel low at about 11 a.m., a weakness which obliges him to take a little something – nothing much, a glass of port, say, or wine with a biscuit. His digestion is slow, so he takes a glass of brandy to help it. His stools begin to be irregular, then there are more serious symptoms: morning diarrhoea which drives him out of bed early, bleeding haemorrhoids, itchy red patches on the skin which soon turn into stubborn eczema. He finds it difficult to tolerate heat. He is always too hot, and throws off the bedclothes at night, because his feet are burning and he needs to put them in a cooler place.

These are the principal indications for Sulphur, the remedy for eliminating autogenous toxins. Sulphur is in fact the basic constitutional

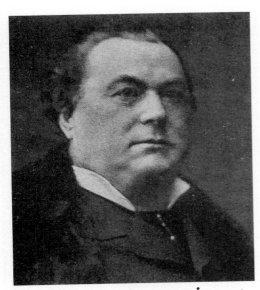

The Actor Dumaine (photo Petit)

remedy of the Jupiterian. It must be understood that all the troubles which beset him – morning diarrhoea, bleeding haemorrhoids, eczema, etc, – are simply manifestations of defence in an organism which seeks to eliminate its autogenous toxins. To treat diarrhoea with an astringent, piles with surgery, or eczema with an ointment will do nothing to remove the cause of the trouble. Indeed, it may do harm by closing the safety-valves which help maintain the balance of the organism. Sulphur acts deeply to ensure the natural elimination of toxins, and will cure the patient's symptoms without giving rise to further troubles. It will help him to lose weight, returning gradually towards the Jupiterian norm.

Jupiterians generally get ill from being too well. They eat too much and too quickly; they drink too much; with age they become fat and heavy, have difficulty in walking and develop general congestion. It was for temperaments of this kind, so frequent in the era of the Sun King, that bleeding became a recognised therapeutic practice. More than one plethoric Jupiterian was treated by this method.

Auxiliary Remedies

The remedies which complete the action of Sulphur, or are indicated in the paroxysmal states which the patient may present, are generally those in the materia medica which gravitate around Sulphur or belong to the same group. To study the members of this group, let us identify the relationships which unite them.

Three remedies suggest that Sulphur will be the next remedy needed: Aconite, Bryonia and Hepar Sulphuris. These are three remedies which can follow one another chronologically, and correspond to three successive stages of the same infection.

Aconite

Aconite is the remedy for acute inflammation that comes on suddenly with extreme violence. Exposure to a cold dry wind is the usual cause of Aconite symptoms. Extreme agitation and anxiety accompany its other morbid manifestations. Think of the Sulphur patient, already congested and plethoric; his healthy appearance, or rather his apparent excess of good health, has led him to believe that he will never be ill. The unforeseen suddenness of feverish symptoms startles him, his usual state of congestion becomes worse; flushed and shivering, a prey to a dry fever without sweating, he rapidly becomes even more agitated and anxious.

Often no diagnosis can as yet be made, but if the precise signs of Aconite are recognised, just give this one remedy and you will be surprised at the rapid results obtained. Often the expected localisation does not take place, and a single follow-up dose of Sulphur will restore the disturbed order.

Bryonia

Bryonia is often the remedy which follows Aconite when a serious lesion exists. The patient's disordered agitation gives way to impassive immobility. The sharp pains of indeterminate localisation of which Aconite patients complain have been replaced by a pain with clear modalities. Aggravated by the slightest movement, it is always improved by

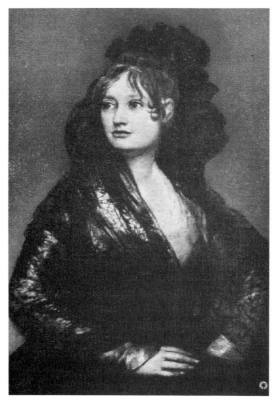

Goya, *Portrait of Doña Isabella Cobos de Porcet* (National Gallery, photo Anderson-Giraudon)

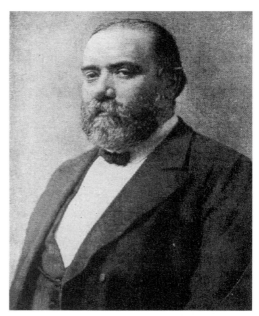

The Critic Francisque Sarcey (photo Frank)

hard pressure and rest. The patient stays completely still, lying on the affected side. The slightest movement causes him to cry out. If you press with your hand upon the affected side or joint, the pain diminishes considerably and the patient is able to move. Bryonia is the remedy par excellence for inflammation of serous tissue and the resulting effusion, meningeal or peritoneal, pleuritic or articular. To hasten resorption we shall again need to give Sulphur, but we shall prescribe it in a form associated with iodine. Sulphur Iodatum 6c given every three or four days with Bryonia will facilitate the disappearance of the effusion and prevent relapse, especially if we later alternate high potencies of Sulphur Iodatum with an appropriately potentised Tuberculin.

The Jupiterian needing Sulphur is a pro-foundly toxic subject. His organism tries to eliminate toxins, and thus he is frequently the victim of recurring attacks of boils. Hepar Sulph. will then be the remedy of choice, especially if the boils are very painful and cannot tolerate the least contact.

Hepar Sulphuris

It is well said of the Hepar Sulph. subject that he is thin-skinned. This expression suits him admirably, for just as the slightest irritation to his skin causes immediate suppuration, so the smallest contradiction throws him into a state of rage.

Aconite, Bryonia and Hepar Sulphuris are remedies of particular value for acute conditions occurring in the Sulphur or Jupiterian patient, such as acute inflammation, damage to serous membranes or pyaemia.

Nux Vomica

Now consider the habitual auto-intoxication of a Jupiterian who punishes his liver without respite. The damage may take two forms. The first includes the results of hepatic insufficiency,

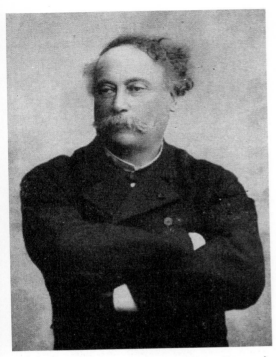

Alexander Dumas the Younger (photo Benque)

If the condition is aggravated, functional disorders give way to more serious troubles. The indications for Lycopodium appear. However little he has eaten, the patient has a sensation of considerable fullness, with eructations accompanied by persistent and intolerable burning felt in the pharynx. The stomach is greatly distended, especially in its lower part, and this is worse between the hours of 4 p.m. and 8 p.m. The liver is painful and hard, and the patient cannot lie on his right side. There is chronic constipation with ineffectual urging; the stools are small, hard, inadequate and difficult to expel on account of a spasmodic contraction of the anus. The haemorrhoids hang down and are very painful. At the same time an alteration of character takes place; the optimistic, cheerful Jupiterian has suddenly grown older. Bad-tempered, especially in the morning, he has become suspicious, talks with vehemence, expresses himself in violent terms and often flies into a rage. Whereas previously he used disciplined words and gestures, now he has lost control; his behaviour is noticed by his companions, who soon become anxious.

which increases little by little, and shows up as digestive disturbances. The other is the result of venous congestion, which similarly appears progressively. Nux Vomica suits those individuals who have over-indulged in stimulants and drugs of all kinds. They are the big eaters whose dyspeptic symptoms take them by surprise. They have heavy feelings after meals, abdominal distension which obliges them to unbutton their trousers, sighs, nausea, regurgitation; the patient does not feel better until he has made himself vomit by sticking his fingers down his throat. Constipated, with frequent insufficient stools, he presents internal and external haemorrhoids which bleed and are accompanied by itching that is worse at night. More tired in the morning than in the evening, irritable and irascible, he is no longer able to work and his intellectual capacity diminishes progressively. It is odd that he feels so much better for sleep – a short sleep refreshes him immediately.

Nux Vomica is an essential remedy for these lapses of Jupiter, which if frequent lead inevitably to the indication for Lycopodium, whose action in proteinaemia is well known. But the venous congestion which often occurs in a sedentary Jupiterian frequently demands the prescription of Aesculus Hippocastanum or Aloes.

Aesculus

Aesculus is a remedy which may be thought uninteresting on account of its limited field of action. It is as ridiculous to say 'haemorrhoids = Aesculus' as to say 'fever = Aconite'. Venous congestion is the dominant note of Aesculus. Everything which increases stagnation in the veins aggravates the Aesculus subject: prolonged rest, sleep, hot baths. He will always be better for cold and for moderate exercise.

Aesculus is a congested individual; he looks

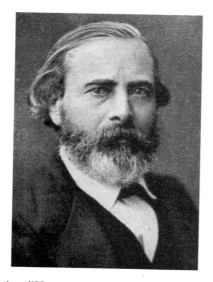

Eugène l'Hoest, *The Painter Edouard Frère*

plethoric and sanguine. He always feels heavy, physically and mentally, and cannot cope with intellectual work; his memory fails and he feels himself to be inferior. This condition disappears if he takes plenty of exercise. Aesculus is always bilious, with a congested liver. The portal congestion from which he suffers is followed by localised troubles in the throat and rectum, whose relationship is easy to identify: the disappearance of pharyngeal signs leads to the onset of intestinal signs, and vice versa. The painful rectum presents five characteristic signs common to Sulphur and Aesculus: burning, itching, feelings of fullness, pricking, and a sensation of soreness; but the haemorrhoids of Aesculus are also accompanied by lumbosacral pain and throbbing.

Aloes

Aloes presents the same signs but without the pricking sensation. The haemorrhoids are very large, very sensitive, irreducible, bulging and hang down like bunches of grapes. The patient has a red face and red lips like Sulphur, but he is very tired and appears stupefied. Incapable of pulling himself together he remains, so to speak, stagnant, with a distended, hot, heavy belly. One other fact is noteworthy: the alternation of headaches, lumbago and haemorrhoids.

Sulphur, Aesculus and Aloes demonstrate well the successive stages of gravity of venous congestion brought on by a sedentary life and alimentary excess.

Consider now the future of a Jupiterian or a Sulphur. Three situations may evolve. The autointoxication of a patient puts him in a state of lowered resistance. It has already been said that serous membranes could be affected (Bryonia), thus pleurisy may occur which leaves no trace. Sometimes the patient even feels much better for it. It is as if the resorption of pleural fluid had in some way immunised him for a while, but this may then be followed by a rapid loss of weight and the signs of Arsenicum – burning pains and the alternation of excitement, depression and physical and mental agitation, anxiety and prostration. Respiration becomes difficult, with asthma at 1–3 a.m., epistaxes and haemoptyses; soon a pulmonary lesion appears, usually at the right apex.

The condition may worsen, and soon the indications for Phosphorus develop, suddenly and violently. A diagnosis is made of progressive tuberculosis, which will need attentive observation and appropriate care. Here again will be found, in an exaggerated form, the signs of Arsenicum and Sulphur – burnings, haemorrhages, weakness and anxiety. But the patient is more resistant. One route of elimination is open to him: the mucous membranes. The destructive process is replaced by yellow, greenish, thick bland secretions. These are indications for Pulsatilla, which parallel the degree of venous congestion. Cyanosis of the extremities, superficial varicosities, varicose veins and dark blood are all expressions of the deep intoxication of the patient. His diminished power of reaction leads, little by little, to chilling of the body, constant shivers, discouragement, timidity and depression. The mucous reactions noted – chronic coryza, chronic bronchitis, leucorrhoea – are not the results of irritation or inflammation, but signs of the defensive elimination of toxins. Here Pulsatilla is considered as a drainage remedy whose efficient action in tuberculinic patients allows the safe use of potentised tuberculin.

With age and excess the Jupiterian grows heavier, his functions slow down, he becomes obese and can no longer lead the active life which formerly stimulated and sustained him. Indifferent, irresolute, and incapable of intellectual work, he loses the taste for activity of all kinds. Fat, chilly and constipated, with a horror of physical exercise, his passive defence against the toxins which are invading him is a crusty weeping eczema with sticky, honey-like discharge. The Jupiterian has already occasionally shown eruptions calling for Sulphur – dry, scaly, itchy, always worse from heat and washing, better from scratching, but followed by intense burning. The lesions of Graphites are better from cold; they are worse in winter, as are those of Psorinum, which in a way is the perfect complement of Sulphur, having exactly the opposite modalities.

Sulphur detests heat, Psorinum cannot stand the cold. The patient is always chilly and wraps up well, even in summer. He is the person with four vests and three pairs of underpants, who never goes out in winter and fears the slightest draught of cold air. This Jupiterian has totally changed, whether through age or serious illness. His loss of reaction is total, and strangely, like Sulphur, he seeks through various channels – asthma, hay fever, eczema, boils, sweats, diarrhoea – to eliminate the toxins, both acquired and inherited, which have been poisoning him since his birth.

Many other remedies are related to Sulphur, notably those which have a centrifugal action on the organism, and which by various routes contribute to the elimination of toxins. The remedies studied demonstrate in particular the paroxysmal states presented by the Jupiterian patient, who is basically always Sulphur.

Life Style

The Jupiterian loves change, and it is important to present him with plans for improving his health that he will adopt voluntarily. Above all, always speak to him with optimism and encouragement. If he is sent to the country, be sure that it is to a pleasant place where the cooking is excellent and where he will be made welcome, because he likes good living and consideration.

If in his daily life the Jupiterian can maintain a discipline which keeps his remarkable attributes in constant activity, then he will remain in a state of magnificent balance. Little food and moderate exercise are the general indications which should be proposed for him. But never put a Jupiterian on a strict diet. Let him have lapses – he needs them. Remember that a good meal sets him up powerfully, not only because of the quality of the food and the wine, but also because of the euphoria induced by happy surroundings and good company. Just tell him not to touch spirits, and not to drink wine every day. He will obey you, because he will rapidly recognise the remarkable influence of your treatment on his condition.

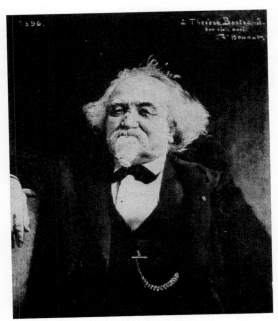

Bonnat, *Portrait of Joseph Bertrand* (photo Braun)

'A good idea must travel through three brains before taking shape. It is conceived in the abstract by Saturn, warmed, coloured and formulated by the Sun, then Jupiter puts it into action, having modified it to the point of possibility. Saturn is the idea, Apollo the form, Jupiter the realisation. Mercury will come along next to adapt it.'

Péladan

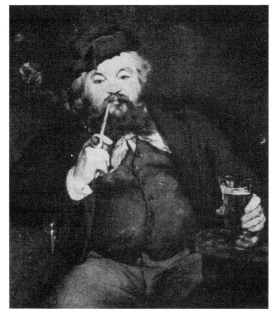

Edouard Manet, *Le Bon Bock* (photo Bulloz)

REMEDIES OF THE JUPITERIAN

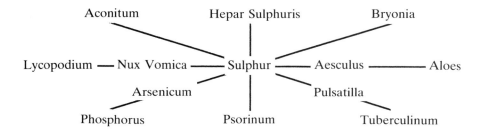

Aconitum   Hepar Sulphuris   Bryonia

Lycopodium — Nux Vomica — Sulphur — Aesculus — Aloes

Arsenicum   Pulsatilla

Phosphorus   Psorinum   Tuberculinum

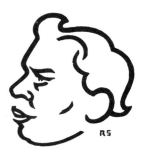

9

Mercury

Mercury is a well-marked Type. Physically he is one of the easiest to distinguish, for his appearance has not changed from images created by artists of old to depict the rapid messenger of the gods. Mentally he has not changed much either, and he is one of the most captivating and interesting types. 'Like the fresh breeze of Dawn,' as Homer put it, 'Mercury, clever and resourceful, crosses the threshold of the house of the Immortals with oblique gait and nimble steps.'

Could anyone paint a better word-picture of this astute and sceptical character whose ever-awakening curiosity touches everything and respects nothing? And when the poet goes on to describe a being 'with slender limbs and wide shoulders', who lies as easily as he breathes, and blocks his ears with his 'tiny hands' so as not to hear well-deserved reproaches, twitching his 'feeble eyebrows' in order to lend his face an

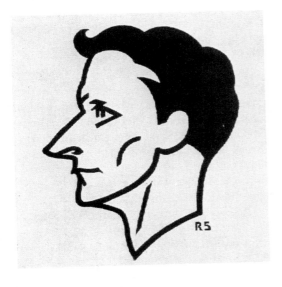

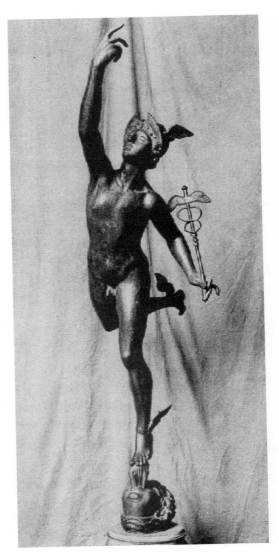

John of Bologna, *Mercury* (Louvre Museum, photo Bulloz)

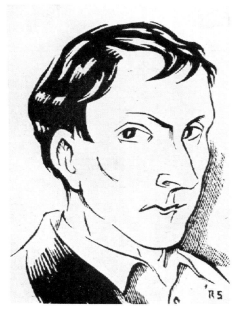

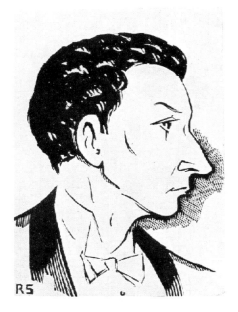

expression of astonishment which his 'misleading but brilliant' eyes deliberately accentuate, who would not recognise the Mercury of our time?

DOMINANT CHARACTERISTICS

Small stature.
Agitated and gesticulating. Rapid gliding gait.
An active and impatient character, inquisitive and witty.

DESCRIPTION

Small stature, 1.60–1.75m. Nervous agitated manner. Rapid gliding gait (walks on his toes). Frequent nervous gestures. Face the shape of a hazelnut. Wrinkled forehead, large skull. Thin straight nose with closed nostrils. Small thin pinched mouth. Rather square slim chin. Small high-set ears. Black hair, which is wavy or curly. Eyebrows somewhat arched and close to the eyes. Sparkling black eyes. Smooth complexion, sometimes with an olive tinge. Thin chest with broad shoulders. Sinewy hairy arms. Narrow hands with tapering fingers. Slender hairy legs. Small arched feet.

MORPHOLOGY

Static

The essential characteristic which immediately strikes the observer is the 'triangular effect' of Mercury's physiognomy, with a large skull and a small chin. This pattern repeats itself in the body, with broad shoulders, thin chest, slight figure and relatively narrow hips.

Mercury subjects are of medium or small build, with slim, well-constructed bodies and slender limbs. Even at an advanced age they have the gift of retaining the appearance of youth.

The face is shaped like a hazelnut, which may be elongated in the more cerebral and nervous Types. The forehead, which has an elegant curve, is high, convex and domed. The nose is long and straight, sometimes a little beaked, but always pointed at the tip, with small, narrow, almost closed nostrils. The eyebrows, scarcely visible, are close to the eyes, and the orbital ridge juts forward slightly.

The eyes are fine and expressive. They are deep-set, black or brown, and always lively and mobile. An important feature, which applies only to the eyes of Mercury, is that they

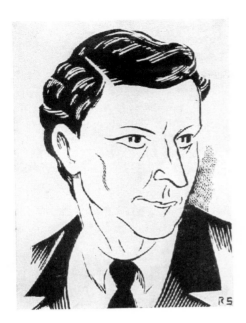

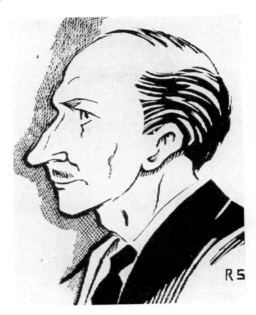

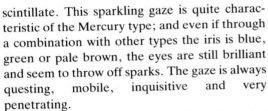

scintillate. This sparkling gaze is quite characteristic of the Mercury type; and even if through a combination with other types the iris is blue, green or pale brown, the eyes are still brilliant and seem to throw off sparks. The gaze is always questing, mobile, inquisitive and very penetrating.

The mouth is small, thin and pinched, but often turns up at the corners. The lips are very thin, but mobile and full of spirit, with a variety of expressions. These are enlivened and animated by sparkling mischievous black eyes which twinkle like stars, giving the face a seductive and original vitality.

The chin is fine and pointed and may be somewhat square. The ears are small and high-set, very well shaped. The complexion varies, but at rest it is usually of a yellowish pallor.

The hair is black, chestnut or brown; very supple, it curls easily, sometimes in ringlets. The neck is long and well-designed. The chest is thin but the shoulders are broad; the back is very straight. The Mercurian woman's small breasts are not round, but pear-shaped.

The waist is remarkably flexible, the loins strongly arched. The slim, strong limbs are small-boned. The hands are very supple, with narrow wrists and slender fingers. The small feet have high arches.

Dynamic

Mercury subjects, both men and women, are young boys at heart and remain so all their lives, whatever their age and sex. Even in old age they retain a slim figure and a mobile, cheeky expression.

Their posture is essentially restless and changeable. It is very difficult for them to stay in one position for any length of time – they need to move about. When trying to stand still, they cross their feet and shift their weight from one leg to the other. They cannot sit still for long, and lose no opportunity to get up and move some object. During even the most serious conversations their hands are constantly busy, tapping on the table or on the arm of a chair.

Their gait is rapid and smooth, as if sliding; they find it easy to walk on tiptoe, since they are digitigrade – that is, their toes point downwards. (Saturnians are plantigrade – that is, flat-footed.) With little quick steps, Mercurians skim over the ground as if they were flying. They walk on the tips of their toes. The Mercury woman walks comfortably on a high Louis XV

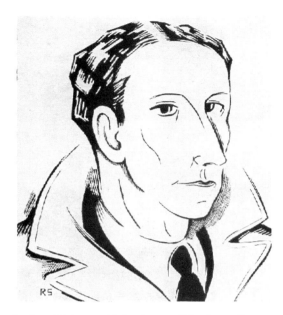

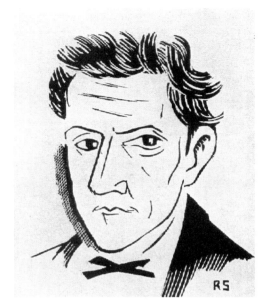

heel, which would be impossible for a Saturn woman.

The instability of their attitude, the rapidity of their gait, the perpetual motion that seems to animate them – all these give rise to the saying that Mercurians have quicksilver in their veins. Their gestures are rapid and prompt, varied and

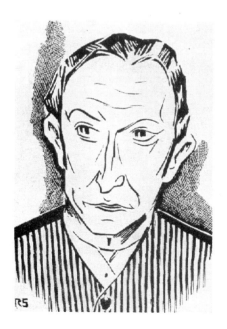

changeable, often bizarre and eccentric. The most striking thing about a Mercurian is his volubility, both in word and gesture. He never utters a word that is not followed by several synonyms; he greets you several times, with his body, his gestures, and his eyes. All his movements are graceful. His liveliness and agility make him a skilful gymnast, and he excels at athletics, fencing and games of skill.

His voice is soft and small. He talks a lot and quickly, in a gay and friendly manner, though his tone may sharpen if he wishes to convince.

FUNCTIONS OF THE TYPE

Mind

The Mercurian is essentially an initiator but he also gets things done. To start a project, make a discovery, launch an idea or build up a business, all these need the participation of Mercury.

Mercurians use a great deal of mental energy, for their searching and inquisitive minds are never still. Their intellects are lively and penetrating; they think with great rapidity. Criticism is their dominant faculty. A sharp, analytical mind enables them to see at once the weak point of an argument or a business, or a machine or a literary work, for they can take on all comers. They have great powers of assimilation and rejoice in an astonishing memory. The spirit of criticism sometimes leads them to sceptical doubts, which they express to the discomfiture of their listeners. Irony can be a terrible weapon in the hands of a Mercurian, but it is never used wantonly. Remarkable for tact, they tease with shrewdness, without seeking to wound their victims. They have a ready wit, coupled with spirited repartee.

In discussions they are not short of arguments, but sometimes they find it expedient to extricate themselves from delicate situations, which they do with skill. Jupiter could not govern without Mercury as Chief of Police or State Councillor.

Energetic, active, with an extraordinary nervous resistance which they sometimes abuse to the point of exhaustion, Mercurians choose to be prudent businessmen, orators who enchant with their subtle dialectic, or artists – above all dramatic artists. As scientists they are very meticulous, pushing analysis to its extreme but then rapidly discovering the means for making a synthesis.

Character

The Mercurian is a sceptic but also a seeker, a progressive man who tries to perfect himself in order to have more courses of action open to him. His inquisitive and curious nature means that he strives to know all, to understand all, to experience all. With a special kind of intuition, he guesses things rather than knowing them, and is able to relate facts from different sources. In everything he is his own master.

The Mercurian has a horror of dogmas and fixed principles; he never believes anything without examining the evidence and acting upon it. It is difficult to deceive him in financial matters, but he is not always scrupulous about deceiving others; he regards it as a ruse, or a matter of diplomacy, and he plays this game like other games of love or chance. He is a clever speculator who really knows the philosophy of success.

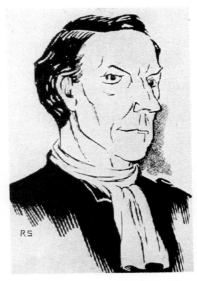

The Mercurian of lower intellect is a busybody who torments his neighbours and upsets his friends by his need for constant activity. He is an agitated neurotic who must have some definite aim in order to use up his energy, otherwise he would set about disorganizing the whole world.

Moderate and reserved Mercurians are not sensual but can be luxury-loving and imaginative, and sometimes go in search of unusual forms of gratification which rapidly deplete their

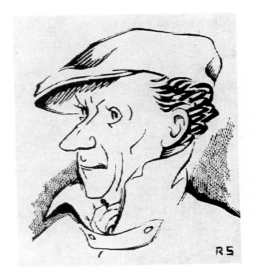

nervous energy, and if persisted in will lead to epileptic convulsions. The ancients depicted Mercury with his male member in full erection. Mercury the violator of nymphs lacks feeling, and his sexuality owes more to curiosity than animal passion. His sometimes morbid desires may have morbid repercussions. Remember that he is the father of Pan and the Fauns.

Lacking in tenderness, yet needing the reassurance of caresses and affection, Mercurians are unconscious egoists; they are also individualistic and ambitious. Their pride goes with a certain disdain for people and things that is apparent in their mocking attitude. Nor do they submit easily to rules or discipline, from which they are able to free themselves skilfully, without a struggle.

They make fine conversationalists, charming, lively and seductive, and attract many listeners; but as their inventiveness is inexhaustible they are carried away without knowing it, amplifying the stories that they are telling with marvellous and extraordinary details.

The Mercurian Woman

The Mercurian woman is always young and always distinctive. Her foot is arched, her leg slim and well-shaped, her waist supple and light, her breasts small, her expression alert, bright and lively. She talks easily and quickly, is good at art and literature, but may be even better as a businesswoman, with a flair for intrigue and all forms of negotiation. In matters of commerce she is often the true head of her household, protecting it where her husband would have let it fail.

She escapes observation because of her rapidly-changing image, and can hide impenetrably beneath an appearance of courtly grace. It is impossible to lie to her, as she is instantly aware of the feelings of anyone who questions her. She detects the secret thoughts of others and does exactly as she pleases, without boasting about it (like Mars), or exaggerating it (like Saturn). She avoids any despotism which seeks to impose itself upon her, escaping from it without a struggle. It is of this type that people

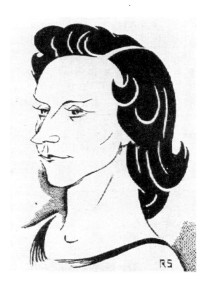

say, 'She would slip through the eye of a needle, and outstare the cat.'

Her memory is prodigious. She never forgets a name, an address, a face or a fact. She knows the history of all the local families, their incomes, and how each one should be handled in order to gain what they possess. Her principle, which could only be that of a shrewd

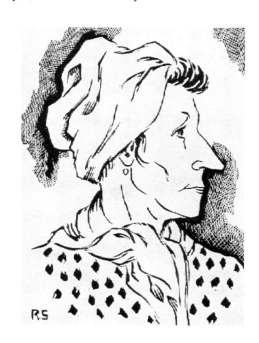

person, is to use the weaknesses of others in order to benefit her own family.

Graceful, a ravishing dancer, and with beautiful manners, she gives everyone the impression that she understands and appreciates them. After Jupiter and Venus, she is the most elegant type. She has a foothold in every world, and her social role would appear to be that of forming a link between people who would otherwise never meet. As a diplomat's wife, it is she who will take the lead in sorting out tangled situations and forecasting the future, for she combines a psychological awareness of people with a strong intuition of events.

DISEASES AND REMEDIES OF THE MERCURIAN

The Mercurian characteristics described above are modified by the constitution to which the subject belongs; they may also be changed by the diseases to which he may fall victim.

Carbonic Constitution

At first it is difficult to imagine a carbonic Mercurian. The flexibility of Mercury presents such a contrast to the rigidity of the carbonic constitution that it is not easy to see how they could combine. But in fact the carbonic Mercurian is essentially a disciplined person. By imposing absolute control upon himself, he knows how to use to best advantage the qualities of speed and intelligence that make up his armoury. He applies to himself the dominant Mercurian quality of criticism; before taking a decision, before even formulating his thoughts, he filters the points for and against through the sieve of his intellect. Thus he rarely makes a mistake, and his capacities for inspiration and realisation can blossom freely.

Phosphoric Constitution

The critical instinct of the phosphoric Mercurian is exercised chiefly at the expense of others. In an inferior type one finds the misunderstood aesthete, the popular dancer, the arbiter of elegance who is the bane of all those worldly starlets whom he dominates so well. A better type is the seer, the visionary who can grasp in a few seconds the strangeness of a situation and predict the outcome, whether natural, artistic or diplomatic. He is the artist who clings to his

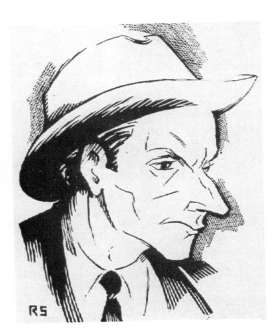

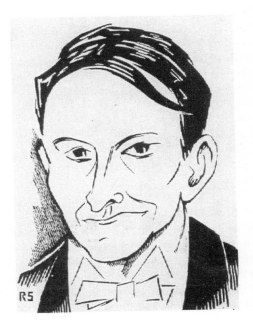

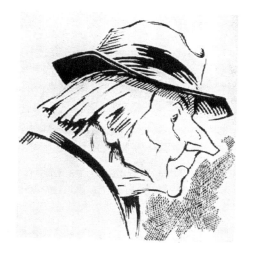

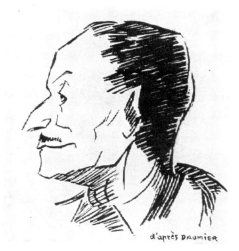

d'après DAUMIER

original vision, even though it may be incomprehensible to his contemporaries. His unconventionality, initially shocking, eventually wins attention.

Fluoric Constitution

The fluoric Mercurian wastes no time on philosophical speculation, for he is primarily interested in money. He can be an unscrupulous rogue who deceives a crowd with his lies. He can also be the skilful speculator who can float a large business with surprising audacity, considering that his decisions were taken after a rapid judgement of certain facts. Traversing the globe in all directions, this is the great financier who lives in a perpetual whirlwind, known and admired by those who are close to him for his intuitive guesses.

TRANSMUTATIONS OF THE MERCURIAN

Morbid Predispositions

Physical Disorders

When he is functioning normally, the Mercurian knows no repose. His restlessness, both physical and mental, keeps him in a constant nervous state. In spite of his stamina this leads progressively to complete exhaustion. The subject then says that he feels 'flat' and cannot do any

more; the dramatic contrast between his habitual hyperactivity, and the weakness and depression which have overtaken him, affects him profoundly.

The major illness of the Mercurian is nervous exhaustion, usually manifesting itself as the loss of all mental energy, with deep discouragement. It can also take other forms that are easily discerned if his functional make-up is known. The constant search for new sensations engenders neurosis, often leading the subject to show neuropathic symptoms such as nervous crises, convulsions and epilepsy.

Finally, it should be noted that Mercurians, even if they do have broad shoulders, also have narrow chests. One result of their constant activity is that they do not take the time to breathe. Sitting in huddled postures they tire out their hearts, which are poorly irrigated by blood low in oxygen. They often experience palpitations and extrasystoles, secondary to inadequate chest expansion.

Despite her boyish appearance, the Mercurian woman suffers from the usual feminine disorders. Her nervousness is compounded by all the symptoms which demand the patience she does not possess. She experiences nervous breathlessness, suffocation, or sudden pains. Because she does not have time to be ill, she collapses for an instant, then starts off again, only stopping in order to die.

Psychological Disorders

The moral malady of Mercurians is telling lies. They either use their mocking wit at the expense of their companions; or else, with the greatest tact, they try to avoid hurting anyone; in both cases their acute sense of observation and understanding of temperament may lead them to unworthy actions. If they lack moral sense they become liars and cheats and fail to keep their promises. They use their wits to the disadvantage of others, even their benefactors and friends. One of them once even wrote to me that 'gratitude is not slavery'.

Their mockery can become spiteful. They take pleasure in venting their sarcasm upon those around them. They denounce and betray people; the anonymous letter is their favourite weapon. The bad Mercurian woman sows discord within her family, repeating to the one what another has said. Bad Mercurians who are in business give false descriptions of what they are selling, and lie about the weight and quality of their merchandise.

Evil counsellors, they incite others to break the law, whilst they themselves watch events from the shadows. They authoritatively affirm the worst lies, the most hateful slanders; they are accomplished forgers who work on peoples' minds with the same ease with which they falsify documents or print money.

Mercurian women often shoplift in the big stores. They do not intend to steal, but find themselves under a compulsion to take coveted objects.

Modifications of the Type

These moral and pathological changes may be observed in Mercurians, whose habitual behaviour is thus transformed and exaggerated. An 'inauspicious' type of Mercury has been described. We should rather call it a 'wicked' or 'sick' type.

The face is distinctly triangular, the eyebrows joined and contracted. The eyes are small, very deep-set, sparkling, snake-like, with darting sideways glances. The pupil is mobile and restless. The nose juts forward and is even more pointed, the mouth, pinched and puckered, is fixed in a grin that conveys both sarcasm and anxiety. The complexion is blemished with many marks. The hair grows in patches and is short and untidy. Movements are quick and accurate, like those of a monkey. Sometimes one shoulder is higher than another. The long fingers make involuntary prehensile movements – a Mercurian avoids opening his hand in greeting.

TREATMENT

Because of his physical and mental restlessness, the Mercury subject who has been overworking is prone to sudden bouts of depression. From one day to the next his nervous batteries will go flat.

Silicea

Silicea is the basic remedy for a Mercurian who has worked too hard and used up all his nervous energy. When he is depressed he becomes childish and fearful and discouraged by the least failure. The depression deepens, the smallest mental effort tires him, and he makes mistakes in his speech. Talking becomes arduous, he seeks for words, and has even greater difficulty in expressing his thoughts in writing. Nevertheless he wants to go on working, even though he has reached the limit of his endurance long ago. He may then be in a state of semi-conscious-

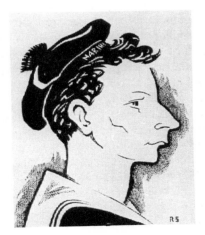

ness, in which his will, already absent, can no longer intervene. He even lacks the strength to stop working in order to have the absolute rest he needs. We are all familiar with profoundly depressed patients who are aware of their physical and mental deterioration, but will not listen when their families beg them to stop and rest. If the doctor prescribes them a cure far from their place of work they may obey with a bad grace, but will be grateful to him later on for having forced them to take the decision.

A wife or husband will take you aside and describe the extreme nervousness of their spouse, who presents a picture of ill-humour and exaggerated irritability. Kept on the move by futile restlessness, he cannot stay in one place and starts at the slightest sound. If a knife falls whilst he is sitting at table, or a glass is suddenly struck, he flies into a temper. His nervous system, overextended for weeks and months, can stand no more. The general hyper-aesthesia is demonstrated by exaggerated reflexes. Often his exhaustion is such that he wants to stay in bed all the time, which particularly worries those around him who are accustomed to seeing him very active.

Another important sign is this individual's increased sensitivity to cold. He catches cold for no apparent reason. He feels the cold penetrating his bones and knows that he can never get warm, yet in winter you will often meet with exhausted Mercurians wearing barely enough clothes. 'It's no good,' they say, 'I cannot get warm.'

Mental exhaustion, moral depression, ice-cold chilliness, a progressive loss of weight – these are the chief characteristics of Silicea which will be found in overworked and 'drained' Mercurians.

Auxiliary Remedies

Mercurians may need other remedies that gravitate, strangely enough, around Silicea. Habitual restlessness is the key to them all – Arsenicum Album, Iodum and Argentum Nitricum.

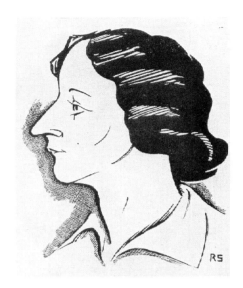

Arsenicum Album

The Arsenicum Album subject presents with a picture of insurmountable agitation, which little by little leads to a state of physical and mental exhaustion. Arsenicum cannot stay in one place, pacing his room or apartment until exhaustion forces him to stop; if he is sitting, he rises every few moments to change his seat; lying down, he is constantly moving about in bed, turning first to one side and then to the other. And if by reason of illness extreme weakness prevents him from moving, then every few minutes he will ask his attendant to lift him up and change his position. Sometimes he even insists on being put into another bed, where he soon begins to complain again and be restless. This pathological restlessness is most marked between 1 a.m. and 3 a.m., and is accompanied by deep anxiety and a dread of dying. 'Well one day, ill the next' could be the motto of the Arsenicum subject.

Iodum

The Iodum subject cannot stay in one place either, and his anxiety shows in an unusual way – when he is quiet and when he is hungry. Iodum is constantly preoccupied, and his worries will not let him sit or rest. He has to walk up and down, whether at home or in the

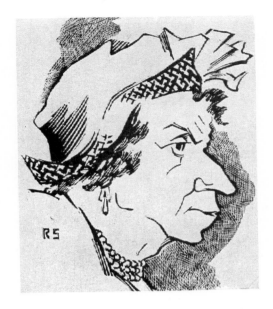

operates at different levels, it is not surprising that his perpetual motion creates a state of disorder. If he does not keep himself under strict control he will also soon exhaust his companions. Argentum Nitricum symptoms are clearly related to the Mercurian temperament: the haste to complete a piece of work, characteristic of Mercurian, will lead him to omit letters or words when he is writing, or to tremble and make mistakes when he is involved in manual work.

Argentum Nitricum needs to do things quickly because he is sure that there will never be enough time for him to finish the task. Time passes too quickly for him and he is always running in the hope of saving a few elusive moments. In normal life Argentum Nitricum, like the Mercurian, walks quickly. The more his mind is disturbed the faster he wants to walk, and he will go on walking, rapidly and purposelessly, until he is tired out.

Arsenicum, Iodum and Argentum Nitricum show three kinds of restlessness that correspond well to the Mercurian temperament. Other symptoms will be found to correspond to the pathological paroxysms which affect the subject.

doctor's consulting room; movement is necessary to him. This restless anxiety is very like that of Arsenicum, but whereas the latter is terrified by the fear of dying, Iodum is anxious because he is worried about his health, worried over unimportant trifles, worried because he thinks something unpleasant is going to happen to him, even though he does not know what, but he always fears the worst.

The feverish activity with which he accomplishes the smallest tasks rapidly leads him to a state of exhaustion which, with his anxious temperament, causes him to lose control of his nervous system. He easily becomes unbearably irritable, with sudden fits of violence and impulses to acts of brutality.

Argentum Nitricum

The Argentum Nitricum subject is perpetually agitated. Always in a hurry, always busy, living with the worry that he will not be able to get things done in time or complete his projects. If he begins a piece of work he wants it finished at once; if he gives an order he wants it carried out immediately. Often, indeed, having given an order, he will carry it out himself to hasten its execution. Considering the increased intellectual activity of a Mercurian, an activity which

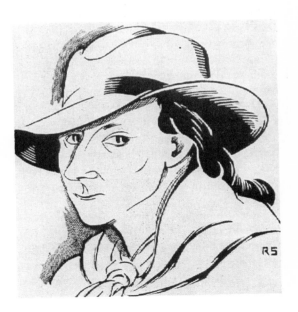

Lilium Tigrinum

Lilium Tigrinum shows a similar anxious agitation. The patient, usually a woman in whom the mental disturbance is related to uterine disorder, is always in a hurry, as if she had important duties to perform which she is quite incapable of carrying out. She is deeply depressed at the alteration in her health, believing she has an incurable disease. She fears being alone, and often shows sudden impulses which cause her to run, to lash out or think obscenities. She complains of pressure in the lower belly that forces her to support her vulva with her hands when she walks. During menstrual periods the flow ceases at night, and only takes place when she walks or makes some other movement.

Lachesis

Lachesis is the remedy complementary to Lilium Tigrinum. Here the agitation is entirely mental, alternating with spells of depression. The patient is exceptionally loquacious, especially at night. She wants to talk all the time, jumping from one subject to another with an incoherence of which she is unaware.

Chamomilla

Chamomilla is a perpetually restless subject who moves about all the time. The young child cannot stay in one place and is exhausting to its minder, who cannot take her eyes off him for a moment. He runs here and there, talks at random, cries, gesticulates, complains, begs, gets angry, and is totally hateful and unbearable. When he goes to bed he will not lie quietly, but struggles, throws off the bedclothes, shouts or coughs in his sleep, and wakes with a jerk, terrified by frightening dreams. He will not calm down or be quiet unless he is carried in the arms of his nurse or pushed out in a perambulator. Amelioration from being carried, or wheeled in a carriage, is a strong symptom of Chamomilla. The passive movement antidotes in some way the active and disordered mood of the subject. In the adult this agitation shows mostly when he is in pain, and is accompanied

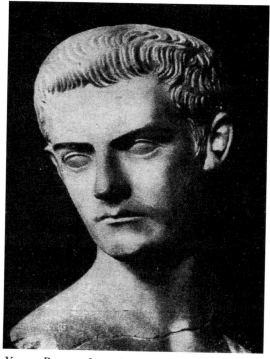

Young Roman, fragment, Augustan epoch (photo Archives Photographiques)

by insane anxiety, an impulse which forces the patient to throw himself about from one side to another whilst lamenting and calling out contradictory statements.

The Chamomilla subject is basically a very sensitive neurotic. His natural instability is not only mental, but physical as well – he cannot bear the slightest pain. (This marked intolerance of pain is seen at its worst in people who abuse coffee.) At the first tiny unpleasant sensation the patient moans and groans; from being merely worried he rapidly becomes anxious about what could happen to him, and soon starts to panic. If he is lying down he throws himself from side to side, lamenting in his despair; if standing up, he tears around like a madman, shouting and declaring that no one in the world has ever suffered so much, calling for death as the only thing which can deliver him from his intolerable pain. He calls loudly for his physician but rejects him when he arrives. Or he

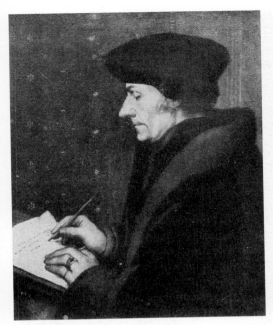

Holbein, *Erasmus as a Young Man* (photo Bulloz)

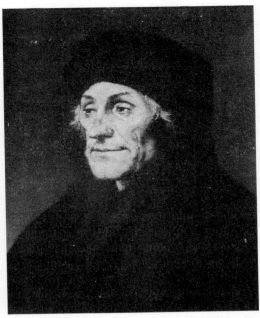

Holbein, *Erasmus as an Old Man* (photo Bulloz)

will enthusiastically accept any advice which may be given to him, and then do something quite different the next moment. Foolish and desperate, incoherent and contradictory, such is the Chamomilla patient.

Ignatia

Finally, do not forget Ignatia, which suits the feminine type of hypersensitivity so often found in the overworked Mercurian. He or she presents with the common vagosympathetic troubles which account for the consumption of a great many more or less toxic pharmaceutical specifics. Ignatia reduces the sensitivity of the subject, and banishes air-swallowing and those other paradoxical manifestations which confuse the physician. The patient is put through many tests, yet all appears to be normal. 'There is nothing wrong with you,' they tell the patient. 'You can rest assured. It's all in the mind.' Little consolation for a suffering patient! Ignatia quickly restores order.

Nosodes

To stabilise a Mercurian one must have recourse to a remedy which can work on the various toxins that contribute to his diminished resistance. For example, progressive loss of weight, paraxodical temperatures, lesions in the lungs or in the lymphatic glands, require the Tuberculins. Increasing weakness with failure to respond to all forms of treatment, total loss of body heat, crises of elimination in the forms of migraine, diarrhoea, leucorrhoea or skin eruptions, call for Psorinum. A history of genital discharge in a sycotic patient suggests Medorrhinum, whose nervous symptoms are well matched to the Mercurian temperament.

The Medorrhinum patient presents a combination of excessive nervousness with an exhaustion that is worse on waking. He is always impatient, anxious, and preoccupied. He has only to start doing something in order to wish that it was already completed. If he gives an order he wants it carried out at once. He only accomplishes half of what he wants to do, due as much to the disorder wrought by his anxiety as

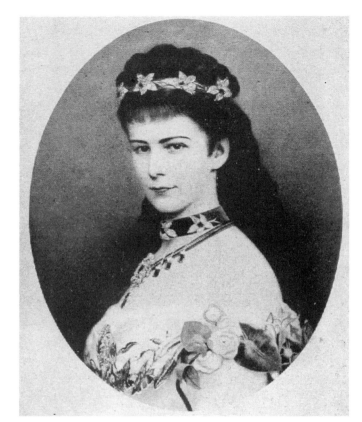

Above:
Elizabeth of Austria (photo Othmar
Türk, Vienna)

Below left:
Willy Jaeckel, *Portrait of a Man*,
(photo 'Deutsche Kunst und
Dekoration')

Below Right:
Jean Mostaert, *Portrait of a Man*,
fragment (Brussels, Royal Museum)

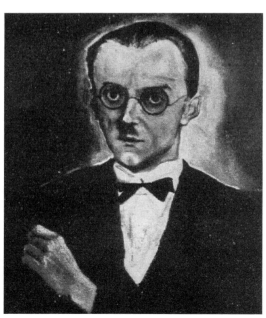

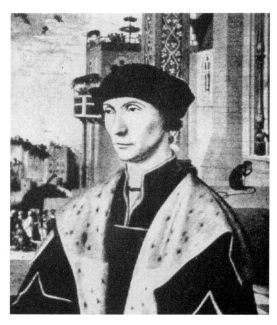

by the exhaustion that suddenly overtakes him. Sometimes he is in such a hurry that he becomes winded and suddenly has to stop, tired out and exasperated by a deep depression. Time passes too slowly for him – in itself a characteristic symptom of Medorrhinum.

Such, in brief, are the principal remedies of Mercurians. We should now consider the way of life that is most suitable for them.

Life Style

Mercury's impatient overactivity can only be countered by more activity. The cerebral agitation he deploys, which quickly leads him to a state of considerable nervous exhaustion, can sometimes be prevented by frequent changes of occupation. The Mercurian must always be doing something, so therapeutic activity should be in contrast with his usual activity. A stay in the mountains will benefit him, and winter sports and summer walks will improve his deficient respiratory capacity. All excursions should be short, and interspersed with stops for rest every hour or half-hour.

The Mercurian cannot stand complete rest. He must be doing something, whether sailing a boat or driving his car. (He should be cautioned against going too fast.) Cerebral overactivity must be compensated for by physical exercise, passive or active – another example of the Law of Similars producing therapeutic compensation.

MERCURY: THE REMEDIES

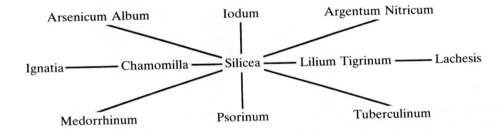

Arsenicum Album — Iodum — Argentum Nitricum

Ignatia — Chamomilla — Silicea — Lilium Tigrinum — Lachesis

Medorrhinum — Psorinum — Tuberculinum

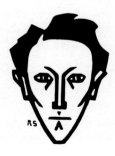

119

10

Luna

Earth's satellite, the Moon, has always been considered to regulate the months and seasons. The phases of the moon were known from earliest times, and the Ancients also attributed to it an influence on the human organism. They had noticed that certain individuals seemed to be more or less affected by it, and that their moral and physiological variations were related to its different aspects: new moon, first quarter, full moon, last quarter. Gradually they came to realise that these subjects always presented with the same signs. But there are different types of Luna, personified in mythology by a series of feminine figures: Selene, Phoebe, Diana, Hecate, Proserpina, and many others. On closer examination it appears that these different creations constitute a number of metatypes, characterised by different associations of types.

Here we describe the pure Luna type, a prototype whose multiple aspects can be considered later. Their variability depends upon the prototype or prototypes with which Luna is combined.

DOMINANT CHARACTERISTICS

Medium height.
Agitated and incoherent manner.
Bizarre, eccentric way of walking.
Imaginative and fanciful mentality.

DESCRIPTION

Medium height. Agitated and incoherent manner. Bizarre gait. Numerous incoherent gestures. Face the shape of a hazelnut. Receding forehead with well-marked arching eyebrows; round skull. Nose turns up at the tip. A

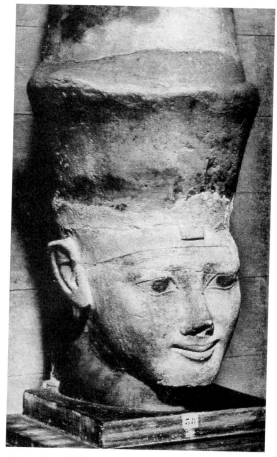

Pharaoh with Formal Headdress, fragment (Turin, Egyptian Museum, photo Anderson-Giraudon)

fairly large mouth which turns up at the corners. Round, short fat chin.

Medium-sized ears with smooth whorls. Fair hair. Lightly arched eyebrows. Blue eyes. Pale, washed-out complexion. Medium-sized bust

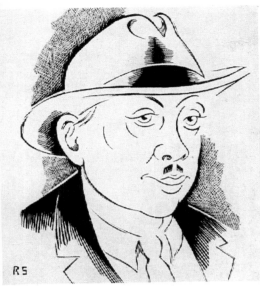

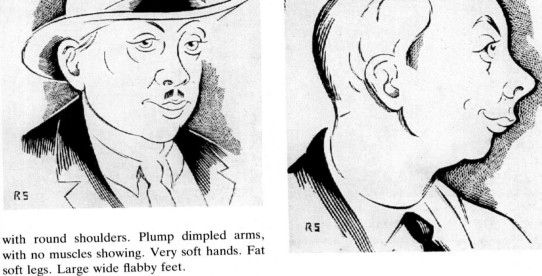

with round shoulders. Plump dimpled arms,
with no muscles showing. Very soft hands. Fat
soft legs. Large wide flabby feet.

MORPHOLOGY

Static

The first impression given by a Luna subject is
that of roundness. Everything about him is
round: his face, his chest and his limbs, whose
poorly-developed muscles cannot be seen. His
flesh is soft; it shows few hollows but many
swellings – which appear when the tissues
absorb water. This often happens in subjects of
Moon type, who are always predisposed to the
hydrogenoid state (von Grauvogl).

The head is round and large above the
temples, and characterless unless seen from the
front. The face is round, and its orb has 'the
shape of a nut'. The forehead recedes gently to
a dome, and is more developed in width than in
height. The nose, short and distinctive, dips at
the centre and widens at the tip. The 'retroussé
nose', shaped like a trumpet with widely dilated
nostrils, is characteristic of the Luna type.

The pronounced supra-ocular arches carry
lightly arched eyebrows, which are very near to

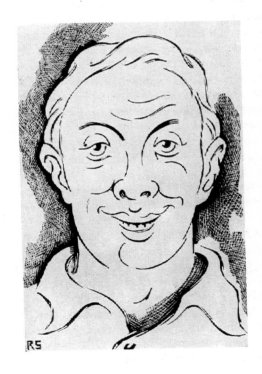

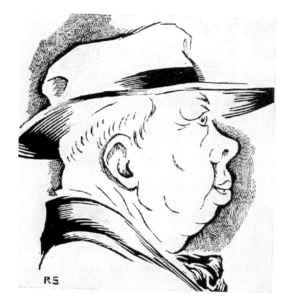

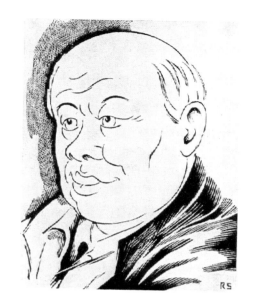

the eyes. The eyes are blue in colour, large, moist and gentle. Round in shape, they are half-covered by big, thin eyelids. The Lunarian, who is almost always short-sighted, peers about in a vague and dreamy manner, as if gazing into the distance. He always seems to be far away, as if pursuing a dream. The popular saying, 'always in the moon', is well-founded.

The mouth, whether small or large, is nearly closed by strong, rounded, reddish lips, whose corners usually turn up. It is typically a smiling mouth, and when the subject laughs it describes a veritable crescent, concave upwards. The chin is round, fat and short. It never projects but sometimes recedes, denoting the passivity of the Lunarian, who is always one to be influenced.

The ears are of medium size, neither small nor large, and nicely shaped, not whorled. They lie close to the sides of the head.

The hair is blond, a kind of ash blond. It is fine, supple, thin and straight – never wavy.

The neck, long, thick and very white, is attached to round shoulders that are large and plump, rather than fleshy. The woman's breasts, slung very high, are small and firm, but they can enlarge rapidly and easily become soft and pendulous.

The back is curved, the waist well-defined,

and the hips are elegantly rounded. The limbs appear to be muscular because they are thick, but in reality the flesh which covers them is soft and fat. The subject often appears to be 'puffed-up' rather than swollen or oedematous; this condition varies with the atmospheric pressure or with the predominantly liquid nature of the diet.

The general impression is of roundness, plumpness and poor musculature.

Kinetic

The behaviour of a Lunarian reflects the feelings which animate him or her. Sometimes, as if driven by an inner demon, he rushes around without pursuing any definite aim; at other times, absorbed by a dream, he remains immobile and sightless in an inaccessibly distant place, completely oblivious of his surroundings. He usually sits with his thighs open and legs spread out, his body bent forward and his hands on his knees.

His gait is irregular and hesitant, odd and uncertain, expressing the irresolution and lack of self-confidence of a Lunarian. He walks with a sense of insecurity, for his balance is far from perfect, and fears he will fall if the ground is slightly uneven. His gestures are slow, awkward

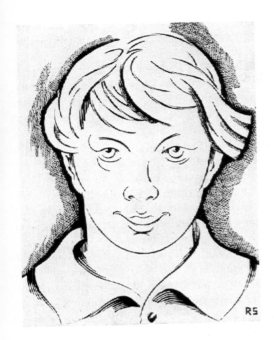

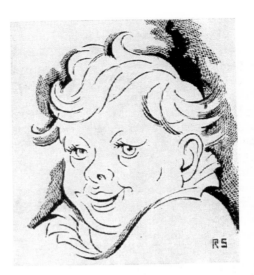

and naive, like those of an embarrassed child. Frequently repeated, meaningless and clumsy, they give the impression that he is absorbed in a dream, or else fearful and absent-minded. The Lunarian often looks as if he has just wakened from sleep.

His voice is soft and agreeable, in a minor key, timid and uncertain. The Lunarian talks seldom, never hums, and in general makes very little noise. His mouth is mobile and variable in expression; one could say that thoughts reach his lips and move them without forming words.

FUNCTIONS OF THE TYPE

The Lunarian has two moods: passive, when he is temporarily under the influence of another person and becomes their satellite; and independent, when he undergoes strange and inexplicable experiences.

Mind

The dominant faculty of the Lunarian is imagination. His inventive imagination works at all levels, but is rarely creative except in poetry and music. The Lunarian dreams, but being un-

practical, does not achieve. He is always in pursuit of chimeras which are not clear in his mind, so that he cannot describe them. He is moved by the profundity of his thoughts; and seeking to recall this emotion may try experiments which are bad for his moral and physical balance. The Lunarian imagination is indeed active. Whether or not he is intelligent, he enjoys vague and melancholic reveries, and will often invent extraordinary stories that have no basis in fact. This taste for fiction can lead Moon subjects to poetry and the composition of reasonably good verse, but also to the wickedness of slander.

The Mercurian lies in order to profit from his speculations, but does not believe in his own lies. The Lunarian really does believe in his, passionately, and affirms the truth of each one that he has related with such convincing ardour. Several months later, or perhaps only several days later, he will have forgotten what he said and will uphold the contrary view. Indeed, he maintains that he 'never said any such thing'.

Lunarians have a prolific and brilliant intelligence. By nature they are intuitive and often have presentiments which do not deceive them. They dream a lot and sometimes have prophetic revelations. Endowed with a remarkable aptitude for poetry, they write harmonious verse with great ease. They are attracted to the marvellous and the fabulous, to paintings of fantastic subjects, like the landscapes in strange colours which are seen in dreams. They like romantic literature, and are enchanted by the works of Edgar Allan Poe. Baudelaire and Verlaine are their favourite poets. Their own timidity prevents them from becoming successful orators, and they write infinitely better than they speak.

Character

Lunarians are impressionable, mobile and inconstant. Always undecided and without much initiative, they have little confidence in themselves. They are alarmed by everything and, beset by imaginary dangers, hover perilously between dread and hope.

They have a horror of conflict, pain and exhaustion, and will willingly sacrifice their own rights to gain the quiet that they value above all else. They are very trusting and thus easily exploited, but bear this fate calmly and with resignation. They are unpractical and cope badly with the material details of life, which in any event bore them to desperation. Anything that requires continued perseverance is against their nature. They lack a sense of continuity and too often allow themselves to be guided by their feelings. They are sociable and enjoy small intimate gatherings, but avoid noisy crowds and formal occasions. They take their pleasure secretly, whether at a theatre or concert or, best of all, on a journey where they are travelling alone or with one close friend – never on an organised package tour.

They like forests, lakes and ponds, taking real pleasure in the groaning of the wind and the murmuring of water. They are nocturnal, sometimes to the point of ceasing to exist altogether during the day; we knew one Lunarian who got up at five o'clock in the afternoon and retired to bed at eight in the morning. They like the night because of the mystery with which it surrounds them, and because of its moonlight landscapes. Moonlight both disturbs and inspires them, whereas they are exhausted and dazzled by sunlight.

Astrology and Astronomy are agreed in regarding the Moon as having no light of her own; she merely reflects the light which shines upon her. Not knowing where he is going or what he wants, the Lunarian is apt to change course without apparent reason, and to desire the things he does not possess. He has a very lively imagination, but lacks sexual drive. Nonsensual and passive in love, he submits to embraces; but the inconsistency of his character prevents him from being faithful, and means that he often changes the object of his affections. His love is idealistic, often attaching itself to an idol conceived in the imagination (especially in the woman Lunarian).

The unknown and the after-life are preoccupations with Lunarians, who have a tenuous hold on life and yet are most apprehensive of death. The Lunarian woman in particular is tormented by strange impulses to suicide.

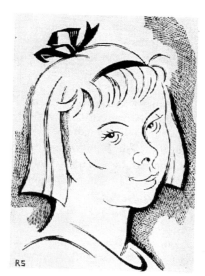

THE LUNARIAN WOMAN

The Lunarian woman can be fascinating from many different aspects. Sometimes pure and pious, chaste and calm, she appears as an almost unearthly being. Many saints were Lunarians; most of them were renowned for their ecstasies,

124

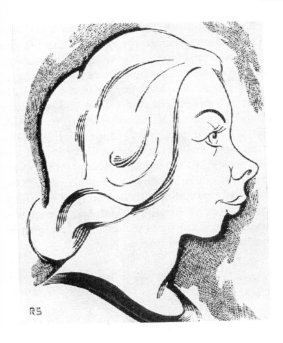
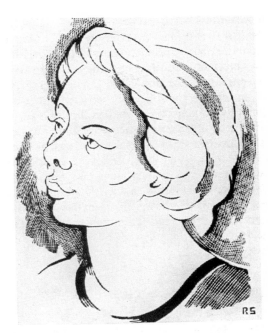

and some for their writings. At other times, excited and rambling, she seems to incarnate madness, crossed by presentiments, shaken by hallucinations and a prey to perpetual emotional agitation. Her nervous reactivity causes her to respond to the slightest stimulus. Attracted by occultism, she readily becomes a spiritualist (if not a witch!). She is a marvellous subject for hypnosis and makes an excellent medium. She is hooked on fear, like a drug. Snow and storms excite her, and she can become intoxicated by a tempest even while it terrifies her.

It has been said of her that the eye is the mirror of the soul. The brighter her eye the greater her sensitivity. If her eye is pure and luminous, then she aspires to an ideal which commands all her reveries and poetic feeling. If, on the contrary, her eye is lustreless – like the eye of a china doll – then this Lunarian lacks all intelligence and sentiment and her imagination will not carry her far.

Always the loser in family share-outs, and cheated in material interests, she offers no resistance to the greed that surrounds her. Her house is Liberty Hall – the servants rob her and the children reign as masters, so long as they do not bother her. She dreams her life, even if she cannot live her dream. She dresses like a privileged creature whose senses are more refined than those of the common herd, and whose imagination is bold and prodigal. Amongst Lunarians will be found women like Egeria, with the gift of wielding strange power over great men. Tormented by wild desires, chimerical and insatiable, they are always complaining and never satisfied. They may become alarmed about their health and suffer from imaginary diseases. The slightest contradiction will cause tears and nervous crises. Anxious and sad, always afraid of compromising her freedom, the Lunarian woman sacrifices her own best interests to her fantasy, attaining no happiness and giving none.

DISEASES AND REMEDIES OF THE LUNARIAN

Before studying the diseases of Lunarians one should be aware of the modifications that can take place in their behaviour, according to which constitution they belong: Carbonic, Phosphoric, Fluoric.

Carbonic Constitution

At first it is difficult to conceive of a carbonic Lunarian, as the characteristics of the Carbonic and the Lunarian seem to be directly opposed. Nevertheless, the notions of law and order so typical of the Carbonic can be found alongside the dreamy imagination of Luna. In this case the dreamer will become constructive and practical. The ideal that he pursues will sustain and elevate him, even if it cannot be completely realised on the human or social level. The carbonic constitution lends the Lunarian a physical and psychological strength which permits him to succeed.

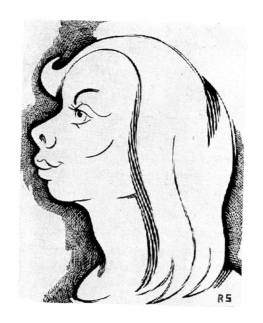

Phosphoric Constitution

The natural enthusiasm of the Phosphoric, and the speed of his perceptions, considerably amplify the intelligence of the Lunarian. His intuition may thus become true clairvoyance. The phosphoric Lunarian is a being who is constantly inspired – his impressions may be translated into exquisite poetry or else into studies in which sublime thoughts jostle with absurd ramblings on the hereafter.

Fluoric Constitution

The Fluoric's prodigious capacity for assimilation is complemented by the natural intuition of Luna, but unfortunately their disadvantages do not neutralise one another. These are well-educated people, obviously cultured and capable of expressing ideas, but they rapidly exhaust their listeners because their thoughts are neither connected nor ordered. The speaker will pass rapidly from one concept to another, but somewhere in this incoherence it will be possible, with difficulty, to detect a dazzling connection. The uneducated fluoric Lunarian is too often a sad purveyor of malicious gossip, devoid of any real interest.

TRANSMUTATIONS OF THE LUNARIAN

Morbid Predispositions

Physical Disorders

The Lunarian temperament is both lymphatic and nervous. Very sensitive to seasonal changes, to the phases of the moon and to atmospheric and climatic variations, the Lunarian is a hypersensitive person deeply affected by his surroundings. We have already observed the morbid pleasure he experiences

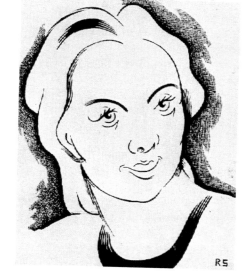

near water, such as lakes or ponds. No one else absorbs more water into his tissues than the Lunarian – his weight often varies from day to day depending upon the hygrometric state of the atmosphere. In fact, the Lunarian corresponds exactly to the hydrogenoid constitution described by the German homoeopath von Grauvogl in his *Textbook of Homoeopathy*, first published in Nuremberg in 1865. (For an exposition of von Grauvogl's ideas, see J. H. Clarke's *Constitutional Medicine: with Especial Reference to the Constitutions of Dr von Grauvogl.*)

The tissues of the Lunarian readily become heavier on account of the excessive water that they retain. This patient does not present with true clinical oedema, but is 'puffed-up' instead. The body shows a generalised swelling, more marked in the face and in the feet. The face may present bizarre variations: sometimes it is puffy, as if the cheeks were blown out, the complexion changing from pink to pallid; at other times it is normal and the cheekbones project.

The Lunarian is subject to intermittent fevers and disorders of the spleen. Lunarian women have leucorrhoea. When they are pregnant they may show a kind of generalised oedema which raises the alarm for anasarca and albuminuria. The poor patient is restricted to a severe diet which she does not understand, when it would have been sufficient to recognise and treat the hydrogenoid condition. Labour is usually rapid and easy, but is often followed by haemorrhage and prolapse.

Psychological Disorders

The moral defect of the Lunarian is 'fantasy'. His actions are always influenced by the caprice that animates him. There is no order in his life, whose pattern depends on impressions received, enthusiasms and irrational exaltations that first lift him up and then exhaust him. We give the name 'lunatic' to a person whose motives are inexplicable and cannot be described in terms of normal psychology. The Lunarian easily becomes a lunatic. Crazy and capricious, he initiates events which could lead to the eclipse

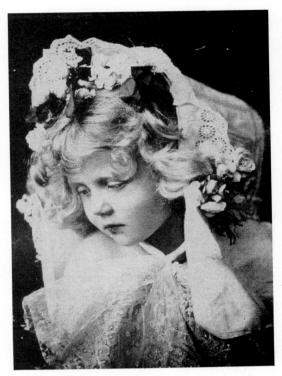

Portrait of a Little Girl (photo R.P.H.)

of family peace. The red moon often destroys the honeymoon. 'To cry for the moon' means to desire the impossible. The Lunarian is often misunderstood, but can also be incomprehensible to his companions, who cannot make sense of his incoherent and frequently delirious imagination.

Uncontrolled imagination without pause or direction dominates the Lunarian. Seekers of new thrills and new sensations, their fantasies will not stop at abominable practices. They consort with unbalanced companions, and will often abuse addictive substances.

They are superstitious, trembling at the mention of an inauspicious prediction, and they dabble in occult science in a superficial way. The female Lunarian is often a gifted seer. In her normal state she already perceives sounds, shapes and contacts which do not exist for others – put her in a trance and she will have second sight.

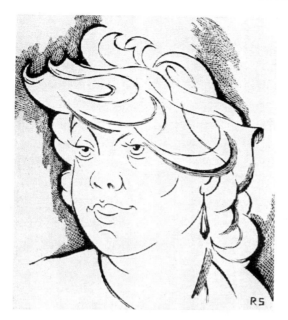

Inconstant and whimsical, and persuaded of the truth of their own lies, they spread disorder wherever they go. Their lack of equilibrium, aggravated by the punishment they receive from their affronted fellow-men, often leads them to dementia or suicide.

Modifications of the Type

The appearance of Lunarians is affected by the morbid conditions to which they are subject. The normal characteristics of the type remain, but their harmonious curves become wider, flatter and less elegant. The face is rounder, the irregular eyebrows meet, the forehead recedes further, and the eyes, always inclined to bulge, project like the lenses of a myopic. The eyeball clouds over, so that the gaze becomes malign and fixed. The bridge of the nose sinks still further, whilst the chin hardens.

The whole body seems heavier, as if thickened and bloated. Massive shoulders support a thin neck. The fatty tissue of the arms separates into lumps; a woman's soft breasts become bulky and pendulous. The thighs become weightier, the ankles swollen, the feet large and thick.

TREATMENT

The Lunarian frequently exemplifies the hydrogenoid state. This can be characterised as follows:

Physiologically
Hydraemia, accumulation of water in the tissues. Too much of the water absorbed is retained, rather than eliminated.

Clinically
A syndrome presenting the following feature: a tendency to swelling, but to puffiness rather than true oedema.

i) The patient cannot remove her rings on wet days.
ii) Increase of weight from one day to another.
iii) Extreme sensitivity to damp.
iv) Aggravation in damp climates, or when staying at the seaside. Aggravation near water, but especially near lakes, marshes or underground water-tables (still water aggravates more than running water).
v) Aggravation from water-containing foods, especially vegetables such as mushrooms, cucumbers, etc.

Basic Remedies

The troubles of the Lunarian are associated with three principal remedies: Natrum Sulphuricum, Pulsatilla, and Antimonium Crudum.

Natrum Sulphuricum
This remedy presents certain dominant characteristics. Thin or fat, the Natrum Sulphuricum patient has one distinct feature – he is puffy. This puffiness extends to the eyelids, the cheeks, the hands, the fingers, the ankles and the feet. It consists of a generalised swelling of the tissues, rather than a true, pitting oedema. The hands are plump and dimpled and become swollen and puffy. The fingers can inflate in a few hours under the influence of the prevailing barometric pressure, and then the patient will find that she cannot remove her rings, and may gain one or two kilograms weight in twenty-four

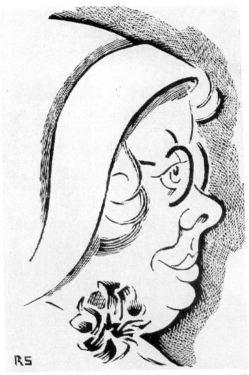

hours. Finally, though the puffiness of the cheeks may be pronounced, it often co-exists with wrinkles and crow's feet at the junction of the eyelids.

The Natrum Sulphuricum complexion is often yellowish or greyish-earthy. This is the patient of whom one says, 'He looks dirty, as if he never washed himself', or else, 'Extremely sensitive to damp'. The symptoms of this remedy are provoked by damp in all its forms – damp climate, atmospheric humidity, damp houses, the seaside; even eating foods which contain a lot of water produces the same effect. Nor should we omit to mention the adverse effect of subterranean water-tables.

'Morning diarrhoea after breakfast.' Acute or chronic diarrhoea is accompanied by excessive flatulence. Preceded by borborygmi and very painful colic, it is at first periumbilical, then following the course of the ascending colon, it makes itself felt urgently after breakfast. The watery, yellow stool is passed in noisy jets, always accompanied by an emission of gas.

'Loose cough with a tendency to asthma.' The cough brings up thick greenish strings of mucus and is accompanied by pain in the left arm. In Natrum Sulphuricum the pulmonary symptoms are usually localised in the base of the left lung. Cough and asthma are always worse in damp weather.

'Left laterality.' The symptoms of Natrum Sulphuricum are predominantly on the left side, and the patient with pulmonary disease cannot lie on his left side. The left base is most often affected. The spleen is often enlarged, with a sensation of weight in the left hypochondrium. Rheumatic pains are more frequent and more marked on the left side.

Natrum Sulphuricum is indicated in the chronic rheumatic patient whose pains are changeable and affected by variations in temperature and, especially, weather. These pains, whether sharp or dull, oblige the patient to change his position constantly. The same modality applies to Rhus Tox., but here it is not the pain which forces the patient to move so much as the progressive stiffness, which leads to a fear of ankylosis. The pains of Natrum Sulphuricum are always accompanied by 'cracking joints'.

Natrum Sulphuricum is also the remedy for asthma which appears or gets worse from

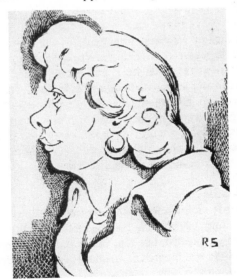

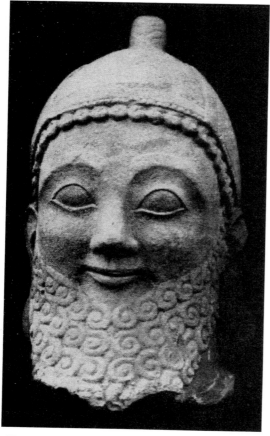

Head of a Man (primitive Greek art, Photo X)

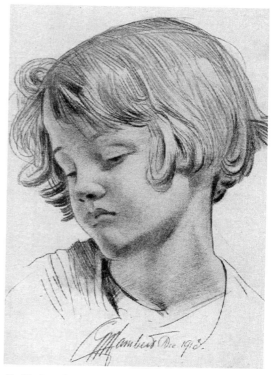

G. N. Lambert, *Portrait of a Child* (photo 'The Studio')

changes of weather, principally at the seaside. The expectoration is thick, stringy and green, the cough is exhausting and accompanied by pain in the left arm. Flatulent diarrhoea which comes on immediately after breakfast, and a tongue covered by thick, greenish-grey coating, complete the picture. You will often find it in Lunarians, especially in spring and autumn when the rainy season begins.

Pulsatilla

The irregular symptoms so typical of Luna call to mind Pulsatilla, changeable, unstable, variable, inconstant. The timid and emotional Pulsatilla will be present to some extent in every Lunarian. Erratic pains which come on sud-

denly and disappear gradually, usually accompanied by shivering without fever; delayed, scanty, intermittent menstrual periods, preceded and followed by thick white milky non-irritant discharge; these are signs which will also be found in the Lunarian. The puffy extremities may show a degree of cyanosis, suggesting a tuberculinic condition.

Antimonium Crudum

This remedy is perhaps the one most perfectly adapted to a Lunarian. Consider its mental (or perhaps one should say psychological) symptoms. In the materia medica the following picture will be found: a girl or young woman who is habitually sad and sentimental, who alternates enthusiasm with crises of nervous depression or melancholia, characterised by the important modality 'Worse at night, by moonlight'. You may meet such a Lunarian, man or woman, and observe their curious reaction to a moonlit landscape, especially if it contains a lake or pond of still water. A sudden melancholy will take the place of the fantasy which enthralled him only a few minutes before. Later you will learn that he is always worse for a cold bath, or in cold, damp weather.

Pulsatilla and Antimonium Crudum are two remedies of great importance to the Lunarian, and Natrum Sulphuricum can be considered as their complementary remedy.

Auxiliary Remedies

There are other remedies to be considered for the Lunarian who is particularly sensitive to atmospheric changes, especially to damp. As soon as it rains she swells up, and often develops joint pains.

Rhus Toxicodendron

This is indicated when there is articular inflammation, or even simply an increase in fluid in the serous periarticular bursae. The patient is restless at night; he cannot find a comfortable

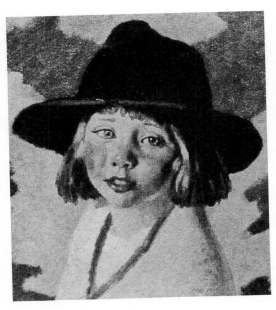

William Orpen, *Portrait of a Child*, fragment
(photo 'The Studio')

position to soothe his painful limbs. In the morning he is stiff and bent, as if ankylosed, and it is only after a few agonizing movements that he can recover his mobility, and even that is very limited.

Rhododendron

Rhododendron will suit those people whose excessive nervous spasms are greatly affected by storms, above all by thunderstorms. As soon as the electric tension in the atmosphere rises, the Lunarian feels upset, and his anxiety will turn to terror when he hears the growl of thunder. And the nervous tension of a Lunarian may take other forms: Nux Moschata, with its changeable moods, laughing or whimpering, gay or serious, lively or calm. This remedy has two essential keynotes – an invincible desire to sleep, and a tendency to feel ill at any moment, brought on by the slightest degree of fatigue or emotion. Note the usual appearance of the patient who needs Nux Moschata – immobile and silent, with closed eyes, as if absorbed in dreams or far-away thoughts.

Ignatia

Ignatia is another remedy frequently indicated in Lunarians. The paradoxical nature of the complaints which respond to this remedy is reflected in the unstable Lunarian behaviour. The pains and functional disturbances, always erratic and contradictory, changeable and unpredictable, which constitute the essential nature of this remedy, are also found in Lunarians. Ignatia will be found most useful in relieving the frequent depressions which follow grief or nervous exhaustion in them, as well as – it must be admitted – the slightest setback.

To complete the list, there are two more important remedies – Dulcamara and Thuja.

Dulcamara

This is a remedy for the hydrogenoid state, meriting a place beside Natrum Sulphuricum, with which it shares several analogous symptoms; but the Dulcamara patient is also influenced by the moon, and it is at the waning of the moon that their symptoms usually appear. Painful enlargement of the cervical, axillary or inguinal lymph-nodes, which comes on suddenly during the night in cold, damp weather when the moon is waning, is a sign that must not be overlooked.

Thuja

Thuja could be the basic remedy for a Lunarian whose emotional hypersensitivity is charged with sadness. In a patient suffering from the effects of a past attack of urethritis, imaginative fantasy can give way to an obsession with fixed ideas, which can be accounted for by toxic changes in the system. He thinks a stranger is walking beside him, or that he is being followed, that his body is made of brittle glass which the least shock could shatter, or – a fairly common delusion – that a living being is moving inside his body.

It is important to note that most of the remedies for the hydrogenoid state are deep-acting and proliferative. In Antimonium Crudum there is horny induration, dystrophy of the nails, painful

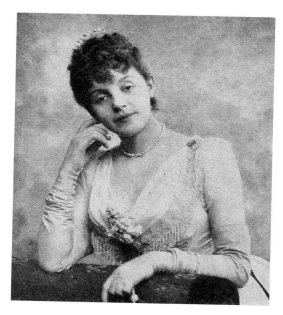

The Actress Réjane (photo X)

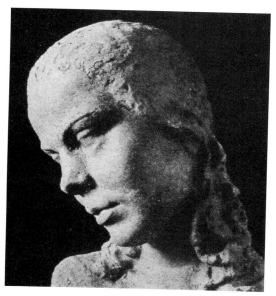

Elisabeth von Esseo, *Head of a Woman* (photo 'Deutsche Kunst und Dekoration')

warts; in Dulcamara, large smooth warts on the face and on the backs of the hands; in Thuja, burning itching warts which are damp and bleed easily, cauliflower-like growths in the genital and perianal regions; condylomata, polyps, all the multiple varieties of tumour formation, from the most benign to the most malignant. Think of the Lunarian as a round person who is predisposed to cancer. We shall then understand the importance of an early prescription of Thuja, and keep watch for the smallest indication that it is needed.

Lifestyle

The Lunarian is physically and mentally irritable. Usually hydrogenoid, he sometimes gains weight very suddenly, when he becomes heavy, coarse and pessimistic. He is full of fantasies and difficult to manage, and it is only by the use of much authority that he can be persuaded to exercise his body and take an interest in his diet. His special signs are that he always agrees with what you say, but the next day assures you that you never said it; and that he begins everything but finishes nothing.

Conclusion

An essentially mutable and inconstant being, the Lunarian is happiest when he can follow his dream far from a humanity that he cannot really see, and which, moreover, does not understand him. His already developed intellect then expands, and carried away by his lyricism, he expresses what he feels and sees. He becomes a magnificent communicator who can translate all the vibrations of his soul into poetry.

More often, alas, unable to rise to such heights, he seeks to exert a malign power over his companions. His life becomes peopled with fantasies and illusions, fruits of his bizarre imagination. He lies, believing in his own lies, and later contradicts them with as much vigour as when he first launched them.

A morbid being, difficult to comprehend, but one from whom it is important to know how to protect oneself. The Lunarian will often end his days in a psychiatric hospital, where he will fade away in a state of melancholia.

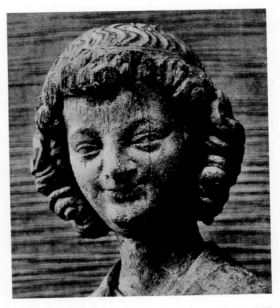

Champenoise School, *Head of Angel*, mid-XIII century (Masterpieces of the Louvre, gothic heads, Editions Calavas)

REMEDIES OF THE LUNARIAN

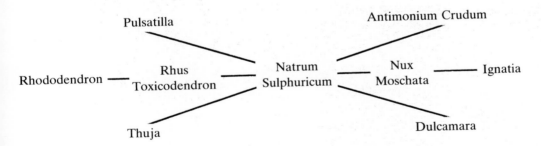

Pulsatilla

Antimonium Crudum

Rhododendron — Rhus Toxicodendron — Natrum Sulphuricum — Nux Moschata — Ignatia

Thuja

Dulcamara

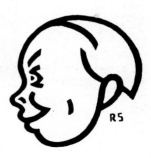

11

Terra

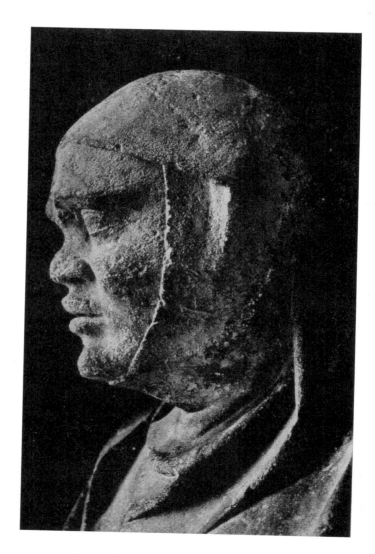

Hooded Man (Champagne, mid-XIII century,
Masterpieces of the Louvre, gothic heads, Editions
Calavas)

Earth is not included in the astral nomenclature of the Middle Ages. Nevertheless mythology, the first science of Types, accords it justifiable importance.

Two concepts dawned upon the human mind from the time man first began to contemplate – those of Heaven and Earth. Heaven is the realm of the stars, whose places in the firmament constitute a guide on the law of the world, to shepherd, sailor, scientist and seer alike. Earth is matter, as Heaven is spirit. Earth is solid, here and now, whereas Heaven is abstract, far away, the future. Earth is mother of the concrete and can only perceive that which really exists.

Seven prototypes have been described. They are like the seven colours of the spectrum, whose combination produces white light. Together they represent humanity and allow an interpretation of it. Would it be wise to omit the earthy prototype whose characteristics appear so often, providing the opportunity of understanding the function of so many human beings?

DOMINANT CHARACTERISTICS

Thick-set, of medium build.
Grave manner.
Ponderous gait.
Reasonable and balanced.

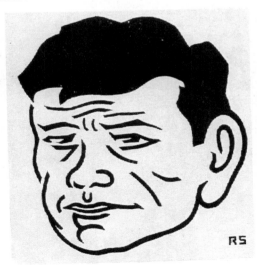

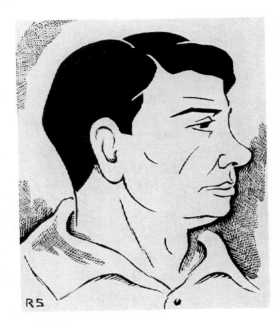

DESCRIPTION

Reasonable and balanced. Of medium height, square and stocky. Heavy manner. Ponderous gait, clumsy gestures. Face the shape of a horse-chestnut. The rectangular forehead is low, broad and flat. Sub-brachycephalic skull. Concave nose. Big, serious mouth. Round fat chin. Large ears with round lobes, like cherries. Black hair. Straight, thick, black eyebrows. Brown eyes. Fresh or rubicund complexion. Short-waisted. Thick short arms, with solid square hands. Thick short legs, with little fat feet.

MORPHOLOGY

Static

The Terran man looks as if he has been assembled from a number of cubes. His build is square and stocky, giving the impression of robust resistance impossible to destroy, of a solid, unshakeable mass. The head looks like a cube. The skull is sub-brachycephalic, with a flat top. The face is almost square, with angular features. Its outline can be compared with that

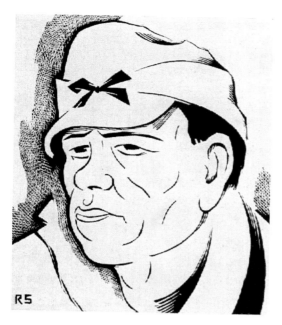

of a horse-chestnut. The rectangular forehead, broader than its height, is low and flat. The nose is quite short, always concave at the bridge, with a swollen, heavy tip; the nostrils are large, and droop.

The eyebrows are horizontal, straight, thick, black and beetling, close to the eyes. The supra-orbital bones are large and jut out. The eyes are deep-set and dark hazel in colour; they often look dull and full of sleep. The upper eyelid is hidden beneath the orbital bone, the lower eyelid is swollen and sometimes violet. The gaze is level, self-assured, calculating and in no way timid.

The mouth is unsmiling, tightly closed and folded at the corners; the lips are ruddy, fleshy and thick. The chin is quite big, usually wide and square, although this can vary according to the associated Type: round and plump for Venus, jutting forward for Mars. The upper jaws are large and heavy; the cheekbones are flat.

The ears are big, with heavy round lobes like cherries. The complexion is fresh, tanned, sometimes reddish. The hair is thick and greasy, deep black, or perhaps brown. The neck is short and thick, carried on high, wide, square fleshy shoulders.

The thorax is short, the waist thick; the chest muscles are well developed in both sexes. The woman's breasts are generous, round and projecting; they are only a short distance above the waist. The back is solid and arched in the kidney area. The thick short arms are not heavily muscled, and the hands are short, square and compact. The thighs are powerful and vigorous, the legs massive, the joints enlarged. The legs are usually short and stocky, and prone to varicosities. The heavy ankle ends in a short, fat foot.

Dynamic

The manner is heavy and ponderous. The Earth man gives the impression of mass that is difficult to shift or mobilise. The woman is of similar appearance, and one hesitates to ask a favour of this robust country person in case she refuses to budge.

The gait is confident and assured, although heavy and ponderous. The carriage of an Earth man or woman can be massive and imposing. Movements are infrequent but occasionally

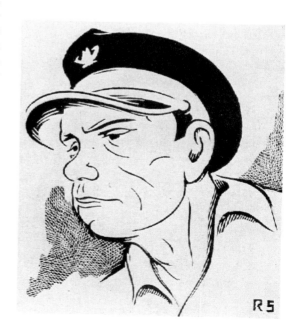

136

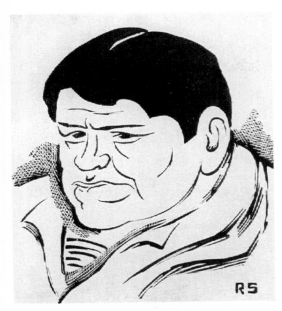

lead to no concrete results. They have a deep perception of the material interests of life, and anything which is not concerned with these is for them idle and sterile. In the field of science they concentrate on facts and experiment. In art and literature they are realistic and naturalistic. In fact, they have very little artistic ability – they look out for that which is solid, good and well-made.

Their great strength lies in the rectitude of their judgement and the common sense that persuades them to lead a worthy life. They have an innate sense of justice and equilibrium. Unfortunately, they assess others from the level of their own intellectual mediocrity, and too often cannot understand the mental functioning of those around them, whom they then judge too severely. The Terran is notable for his capacity for doing nothing. He can sleep all the time, without remembering anything of what has been said to him.

sudden. Terrans are abrupt in their manner – sometimes unintentionally rude, especially if they are carried away by indignation. The voice is loud and emphatic and almost always harsh. It is typical of Terrans to fall asleep as soon as they stop moving about. This is why they often look sleepy-eyed.

FUNCTIONS OF THE TYPE

Mind

The dominant faculty of a Terran is 'common sense'. Reason seems to guide all their actions. They are uncomplicated, sensible people. They do not aspire to enthusiasm, inspiration or intellectualism. They have poor imagination and lack vivacity. They do not lose themselves in daydreams – indeed, they are incapable of doing so. But they are patient observers and seek above all profit and usefulness, everything that will gain them solid advantage. From an intellectual point of view, they might as well be ruminants.

They know nothing of abstract speculation and would not understand it if they did. For them it is a waste of time to engage in philosophical discussions, since these would

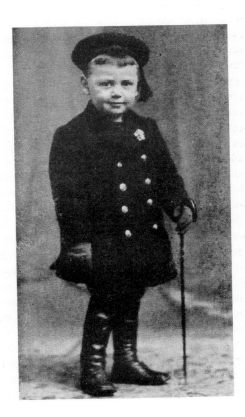

Character

The Terran is both severe and virtuous. He is strict with himself; why should he indulge others?

Terrans are not concerned with the formalities or conventions of society. Without meaning any harm, they offend and annoy people around them, even those whom they love and esteem the most. If they want to be amiable and gracious they do it clumsily, a bit like the Anacardium patient whose behaviour seems to be inspired at one moment by an angel and at the next by a devil. Prone to eccentricity and fits of ill humour, especially when their daily tasks are interrupted, their relationships are sometimes difficult and disagreeable. Nevertheless they are good, in a rough and loyal way. Although they have little understanding of sentimental flirtations or games of the heart, they have a deep fund of compassion which shows itself through their actions. Anyone who asks for their advice after making a mistake will certainly be scolded roughly and lectured, but will also be put upon the right track, encouraged, and often helped – in the same abrupt way.

Patient observers, dedicated workers, they stick tenaciously to their plans and do a lot more than they talk about. They are orderly in business and keep their promises faithfully. But woe to anyone who cheats them! Their anger is controlled and slow to develop, but when it explodes it is terrible. Any decision reached is final, for they cling to the memory of offences and are slow to forgive.

They are true conservatives, motivated by the one idea of improving their material condition – sedentary, attached to their hearth, their home and their country. Whatever their position in life, they reached it by hard work, patience and economy. It hurts them to give or spend money too often. If they continue to withdraw into themselves they become avaricious – like the peasant who increases his land-holding to benefit his heirs, living a miserable life guarding the coins he has amassed, proud of being able to leave a signficant inheritance to his children.

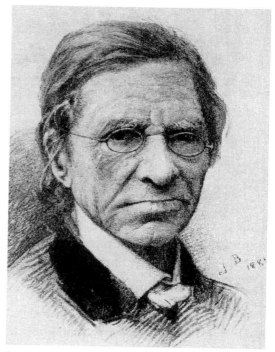

Charles Baude, *Emile Littré* (portrait engraved in France, Editions Calavas)

The Terran is always a peasant at heart. He enjoys country life and work. Whatever his social status he likes to take care of the garden, and is happy to be seen wielding a spade or a rake.

THE TERRAN WOMAN

The Terran woman is first and foremost a good housewife, very economical, and with a perfect understanding of how to run her business and her home. Domestic matters are well supervised and there is no waste. She is a good mother who breast-feeds her children and brings them up well, if rather too severely.

Terran women enjoy exercising authority and giving orders; they resent having to obey anyone, even their husbands. Secretly they are jealous of men, envying their sexual supremacy. With other women they are proud, haughty and disdainful, whereas with men they enjoy an

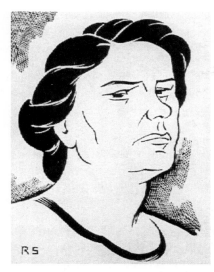

almost light-hearted comradeship and familiarity. Brave and hardworking, and devoted to their family, they are shrewd at business, so long as they are not led into financial speculation. They have qualities which make for success in running enterprises such as a farm, hotel, restaurant – jobs which usually demand the authority and firmness of a man.

One amusing aspect of the Terran woman is that when she has to leave home for an outing or a journey, she at once remembers a number of things which have to be done before she goes.

DISEASES AND REMEDIES OF TERRANS

Before studying the diseases of Terrans and the remedies best suited to them, it is necessary to understand the modifications that appear due to the constitution of the subject – Carbonic, Phosphoric or Fluoric.

Carbonic Constitution

Terrans in their normal state already show carbonic characteristics – stiffness of attitude, monotonous gestures that are slow and restricted. A carbonic Terran creates the impression of a heavy compressed mass, difficult to move, and very resistant by virtue of its solidity.

He does not talk – he acts; he never seeks amusement, working ceaselessly and in an orderly fashion. Hard on himself, persistent in his efforts, he is often stubborn and sometimes quite immovable, although always honest.

Phosphoric Constitution

It is difficult to imagine a phosphoric Terran; the two concepts seem to cancel one another out. In truth, the phosphoric Terran is a fragile subject who has to take care of himself. He must be made to understand that he cannot safely undergo prolonged strain, and that he must limit his activity in order to avoid the depressions that lie in wait for him and which could overwhelm him. He must resist the temptation to rush into projects which fire his enthusiasm, and be persuaded that he needs long periods of rest to restore his balance.

Fluoric Constitution

Every Terran is by nature economical, never prodigal. The fluoric Terran is a miser and thinks only of making money. He will exhaust himself to amass sums that may be quite considerable, and from which he will derive no personal pleasure. The fluoric Terran woman is the old rag-and-bone woman who lives in a shanty and dies on a mattress stuffed with banknotes.

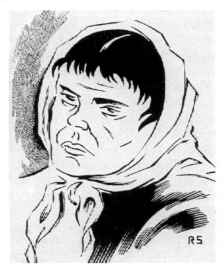

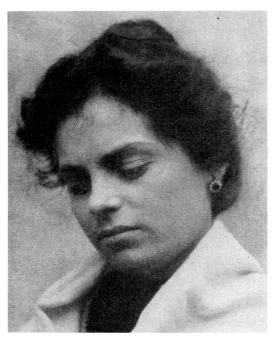

Neapolitan Woman (photo Prof. A.C. and E.R.)

TRANSMUTATIONS OF THE TERRAN

Morbid Predispositions

Physical Disorders

The Terran is a robust subject who looks as if disease could take no hold over him. But he is a short, solid individual, whose organs must be tightly packed into his thickset frame. His life is sedentary, and although he is capable of hard physical work, his movements are stereotyped and do not exercise all his muscles to their fullest extent. He often adopts a hunched-up posture; his breathing becomes difficult, and his heart tires from lack of circulation. Attacks of asthma and cardiac irregularities occur.

Digestive disorders, too, are common in the Terran who fails to look after himself. He may eat too much in order to overcome fatigue. Dyspepsia and enteritis lie in wait for him and lead to hepatic insufficiency. The ensuing auto-intoxication provides the conditions leading to cancer.

His sedentary life is associated with a craving for sleep. As soon as the Terran breaks off from his usual work, or sits or lies down, he goes to sleep. This sleep does not refresh him, but actually makes him more stuporous by diminishing still further the elimination of toxins from his system.

Psychological Disorders

The course of illness in a Terran is related to the failure – or sometimes to the exaggeration – of his responses. His moral malady is discouragement. A shock or bereavement will cause a formerly patient, courageous and hard-working man to become sad and run-down. He will brood over his setbacks in the same way as he used to ruminate over his prospects and plans. If formerly open-hearted he will now be hypocritical and reserved. Whereas beforehand his habitual composure was only disturbed by indignation, now he gets angry for no reason and may attack his family with appalling brutality. If he has been contradicted, molested or cheated, the craving for vengeance gives him no relief. He can become hard and pitiless, and eventually criminal.

Modifications of the Type

Physical and psychological disorders profoundly alter the normal appearance of a Terran, showing the way in which he has changed.

The head is hunched down between the shoulders, the dome of the skull is low, the forehead flattened and crossed by deep lines. The untidy black eyebrows often meet in the centre and are very thick, straggling over greenish eyes of dark and ferocious intensity. The lower eyelids are swollen and look like pockets. The tight mouth grimaces, the chin juts forward, the complexion is earthy, the voice raucous. The arms are large and muscular, with big hands and knotty fingers. These Terrans are hairy and very dirty, and exhale a nauseous odour. Their general appearance is sinister and repulsive.

TREATMENT

The digestive disorders that afflict Terrans primarily suggest Nux Vomica. Remedies such as Lycopodium and Sulphur may be indicated later, but Nux Vomica should always be prescribed first, as its characteristics are the ones most frequently to be found.

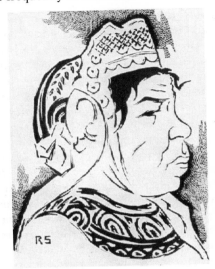

Nux Vomica

The Nux Vomica subject has a difficult digestion. After meals he is heavy and somnolent, and so distended that he has to undo his trousers. He has eructations, pyrosis and regurgitation. To relieve himself of these sensations, which prevent him from working or even moving, he may make himself vomit and at once feels better. Constipation is the rule, with urgent but inadequate calls, and if the patient passes a stool he has the feeling that the bowel is never quite emptied. He suffers from painful internal haemorrhoids that bleed copiously during stool and which are relieved by the application of cold water compresses. This condition is accompanied by constant bad humour which is present on waking and gets worse after meals. The Terran, always anxious to do well, is irritated if he cannot work, and rapidly becomes irascible. Only sleep can calm him. It is noteworthy that a short sleep will produce immediate improvement in the Nux Vomica subject; this is not always the case with the Terran.

Congestion of the liver, which so often accompanies the digestive troubles of the Terran, can worsen and become chronic, taking one of two forms:

Sepia

Portal congestion becomes worse; the attacks, previously intermittent, give way to a constant condition, with the patient suffering continuously from a tender liver. The deep pain he experiences is better if he lies on his right side. Constipation is accompanied by a feeling of a heavy weight in the rectum, as if the intestine was always full. The stools are small and difficult to pass, and there is often the complaint of a sudden sharp pain in the anus, together with an almost constant ooze. There are the objective signs which indicate hepatic disorder – yellow patches across the bridge of the nose, yellow and brown patches on the skin of the belly, shoulders and back, red sand in the urine. A *B. Coli* infection will often be superimposed on this condition; the patient then has diarrhoea if he drinks milk, and cystitis, with frequent calls to urinate.

A radical change takes place in his mood. He

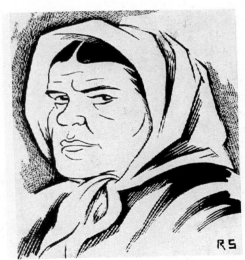

becomes sad and downcast, barely responding to questions put to him, but at the same time is irritable. If a well-meaning person demands an answer, he will show an indifference that gives concern to all those around him. He neglects his business and takes no further interest in the family, even if they had been dear to him before.

Lycopodium

Here the picture is different. The gastric symptoms which called for Nux Vomica have altered. This patient can no longer absorb any food. After eating only a little he is full and distended, but nevertheless still hungry. He even gets hungry during the night, and has to get up to take a snack, such as a biscuit or a little soup. Like Nux Vomica he suffers from pyrosis and eructations. There is the added characteristic, which belongs only to Lycopodium, that the eructation is incomplete and accompanied by intolerable burning which may last for hours, and is felt in the pharynx. The patient complains of 'burning' or of 'hot irons'. Then the abdominal distension increases even more,

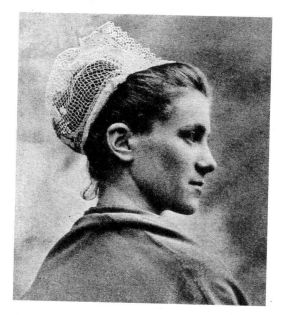

Young Breton Woman (photo Villard, Quimper)

affecting chiefly the lower abdomen, and is worse from 4 p.m. until 8 p.m. The liver is heavy and painful and the patient cannot lie on his right side. Constipation is the rule, with incomplete evacuations of small, hard, gritty motions, difficult to pass because of a spasmodic contraction of the anus. The liver is altered – no longer simply congested – and this alteration is often the consequence of the patient trying to facilitate his digestion with spirits or well-laced coffee. One objective sign is a yellowish face, or yellow patches over the temples. Psychologically the patient is irritable and suspicious, easily loses his temper and uses violent and abusive language; but he is also profoundly discouraged, since he has lost all confidence in himself, and fears responsibility.

Other Remedies

Nux Vomica, Sepia and Lycopodium are the three main remedies for the Terran, but to these must be added Sulphur, the great eliminator of poisons from the organism and the leading remedy for autointoxication. Regular administration of this remedy every fortnight or every month would save much trouble for our subject, who has a great tendency to hoard up autogenic toxins in his system. Remember the chief characteristics of Sulphur – morning tiredness which gets worse at 11 a.m., a constant desire to be cool and breathe fresh air, feet that burn at night and need to be uncovered, urgent diarrhoea at five o'clock in the morning, burning pains, brilliant red lips, and the alternation of skin eruptions with other symptoms. Frequent 'symptom shift' means that the subject never feels really well.

Hepar Sulphuris is often indicated in skin eruptions, boils or eczema. There is a constant tendency to suppuration, every little scratch festers and the patient often has abscesses. He is said to have a 'sensitive skin', because frequent systemic infections cause him to be peevish and feel angry for no reason.

Baryta Carbonica and Opium are useful in the treatment of hypertension, which is common in the Terran.

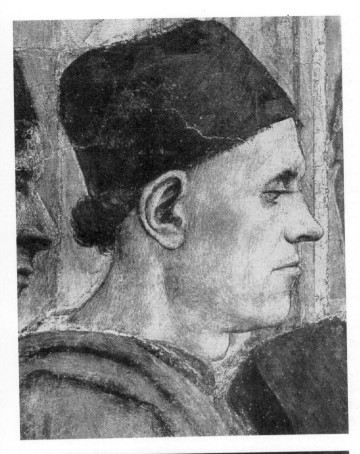

Filippo Lippi, *Florentine Personage*
(Florence, de Carmine church,
photo Anderson-Giraudon)

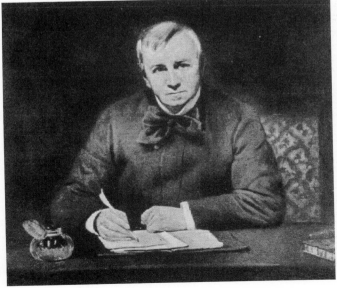

Carolus Duran, *Emile de Girardin*
(Lille Museum, photo Cie des Arts
Photomécaniques)

Opium is particularly suited to the Terran who is habitually congested and somnolent. His face is swollen, red, hot and covered with sweat, whilst his extremities are cold. His head feels dull and heavy, and he complains of vertigo. He sleeps badly; his bed feels so hot that he lies awake and tries to throw off the bedclothes. Bit by bit the congested condition worsens and soon there will appear the signs of imminent apoplexy.

Baryta Carbonica is another remedy for hypertension, but whereas Sulphur and Opium patients are always aggravated by heat and seek the open air and coolness, the Baryta Carbonica patient is chilly. The slightest exertion exhausts him and makes him want to sleep; this is an exaggeration of the habitual somnolence of the Terran. The face is pale, the arteries atheromatous and hard, and the blood pressure raised.

Life Style

The Terran is strong and calm, just and reasonable. You will never have any trouble with him, but neither will you be able to change his attitude to work. The peasant will listen with half an ear to your counsels of moderation, for he knows well – better than you – what needs to be done and what he *must* do. He always finds himself fully occupied, whether he is in the fields, or in his workshop or office. Unfortunately he does not monitor his diet but eats at all hours, claiming that when one works as hard as he does it is necessary to be well-nourished. He drives his car carefully – which is just as well, because his reflexes are far from brisk.

Conclusion

It must be understood that a pure Earth type is very seldom encountered. The functional play of any subject varies with the prototypes with which he is associated. In ancient mythology three aspects were described:

Ceres – the cultivated earth which feeds man as a reward for his labours.

Cybele – the wilderness of sharp thorns and cunning traps; or Rhea, the savage land which defends itself.

Vesta – the deep earth which cherishes fire at its heart.

Amongst humans three types of Terran woman can be distinguished:

The robust countrywoman, the fertile wet-nurse, or the comely shopkeeper – Ceres.

The comedienne, the woman who has her price, the adventuress – Cybele.

The practical woman who watches the hearth and the food cooking on it – Vesta.

REMEDIES OF THE TERRAN

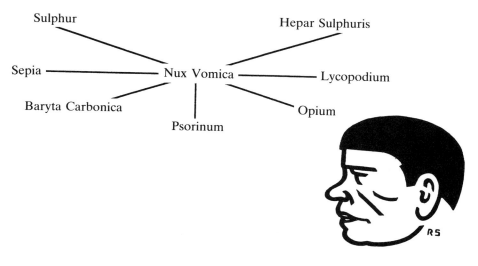

Sulphur
Hepar Sulphuris
Sepia — Nux Vomica — Lycopodium
Baryta Carbonica
Opium
Psorinum

METATYPES

Eight prototypes have been described as exactly as possible: Mars, Saturn, Apollo, Venus, Jupiter, Mercury, Moon and Earth. It is very rare that a pure type is met with in modern society. True, you will often be struck by the physical or functional signs of a type; but do not jump to conclusions – continue to observe. You will soon recognise, superimposed upon this predominant type, two or three types which appear to be secondary, but whose presence in the drama favourably modifies the behaviour of the individual in question. It is difficult to establish a classification of metatypes without running the risk of creating artificial disorder, in attempting to show the different combinations which can occur.

This work owes a great deal to the study of Greek mythology, which was really the first typological classification of humanity. The myths surrounding the actions of the Olympian gods can be regarded as a list of the happenings to be expected in the lives of particular types; or, put more strongly, an exact expression of the function of a god created in the image of a particular man.

Ancient art is no less interesting. The works of Greek sculptors attribute to each type its own structure and character. Apollo can always be distinguished from Jupiter, Venus or Diana. The face may or may not be shown in detail; revelation is sometimes deliberately incomplete, so that the mystery may be preserved.

12

Minerva
(Mars, Jupiter, Luna)

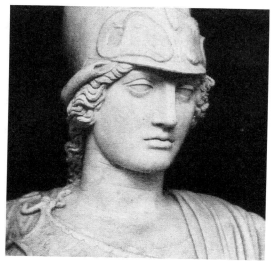

Minerva (Vatican Museum, photo Anderson)

Mythology has it that Minerva entered the world fully armed, with warlike attributes and masculine qualities. Carried in the skull of her father, Jupiter, she was not borne by a mother and never tasted human milk.

Listen to the words of Vulcan as he addresses Jupiter in the *Dialogues* of Lucian: 'It is not surprising, O Jupiter, that you were irritable, whilst you carried, wrapped in your cerebral membranes, a live young woman of such a size, armed from head to foot. Watch her dance the Pyrrhic Dance, shake her shield, brandish her lance, full of enthusiasm. Indeed, she was born nubile and beautiful, in spite of her sea-green eyes.'

Glaucopis Athene was the name given by the ancients to Minerva of the sea-green eyes. They are really the green eyes of Mars, modified by the bluish tint of Luna and the hint of light yellow in Jupiter's iris.

DESCRIPTION

Mars, Jupiter, Luna. These are the components of the metatype Minerva.

Her cheeks are brick-red, blood-red or deep rose, according to which type is dominant. Her hair is warmly coloured: chestnut, rusty or brown. Her forehead is domed. The nose is aquiline, slightly hooked. Her eyes are sea-green. Her mouth is shaped like a bow, with strong jaws and full cheeks. The chin is large and firm. Her neck is strong, her chest well-developed, with firm flesh. Her figure is braced, her limbs solid.

She is naturally majestic and does not seek to be otherwise. Minerva is sure of herself, haughty, implacable and vindictive, but can show tenderness towards a weaker being. She is a typical masculine woman.

FUNCTION

Her dominant qualities are energy and reason. Her moral malady is anger and a tendency to lose her temper. Minerva is an interesting character to observe. At first she may appear to be unbalanced, but subsequent events demonstrate that her actions were reasonable. Bold and audacious, active (perhaps excessively so), a fantastic warrior; impulsive and vindictive, but at the same time generous. She never retreats, as is shown in the following story:

The warrior goddess struck the earth with her spear. Immediately there sprang up an olive tree bearing fruit – the symbol of peace. In a

146

dispute with Neptune over the sovereignty of the city of Athens, she demanded a plebiscite. All the men voted for Neptune, all the women for Minerva. But the number of women exceeded that of men – by one, so Minerva triumphed. She then raised an altar to forgetfulness – and was reconciled with Neptune!

Meanwhile she happily undertakes women's work, and claims to be better than even the best craftswoman. Her vanity allows her to brook no rival, and it was only too easy to turn Arachne into a spider. Her mind is full of contradictions: impetuous, ardent, imaginative, but able suddenly to apply herself calmly to a quiet task.

Minerva is a natural feminist, from an inner need for militant activity. She is not always a lovable woman, but she is well-meaning, and if she were not hindered in her activities by physical disorders or by inopportune sympathies she would be invincible. She controls the lightning, she brings victory, she creates her own strategy, she brandishes her shield, deliberately flaunting the head of the Gorgon Medusa. She is lofty, pure Thought – less abstract, less absolute, less fleshless than the thoughts of Saturn, but more lively and up to date. She is the Intelligence which guards the city. She is National Opinion. This is why Jupiter produced her armed and armoured. We see her as a young girl with a high forehead and a clear and steady gaze, who presides, active but thoughtful, over the feminine arts and the intellectual life of the city. If war should come, hers will be the helmeted head which claims victory, even at the cost of supreme sacrifice.

Metatypes of Minerva

A Marsian type – Bellona.

A Jupiterian type – because she was born of Jupiter.

An Apollonian type – because she is clever and artistic.

A Lunar type, with azure eyes. In her statues, the metal composing the eyes has a bluish tinge.

13

Pallas
(Saturn, Mars, Mercury)

Pallas is a type of woman with masculine qualities, but without subtlety.

DESCRIPTION

Tall stature. Black hair. Long face with strong features. Hooked nose. Very sharp, very black eyes. Chin like a boot (Mars) or like a horse (Saturn). Long stiff neck. Long legs supporting a narrow, flat torso which is held stiffly to attention.

FUNCTION

Dominant qualities: logic and deduction. Moral malady: pride and arrogance.

Pallas is tough, busy, insensitive and arrogant. She knows exactly what she wants. She is an implacable logician, a tactician of the first order, the warrior goddess of Reason. Analytical, meticulous and deductive, her mind turns to dogmatic and authoritarian scepticism. Unfortunately, though her constitution is powerful and resistant, organic weakness sometimes breaks her will. She is subject to fainting attacks provoked by circulatory and nervous disorders, the consequences of a violent temperament and a nature overstretched by the constraints which pride imposes on her. She sobs when she is alone, blushes if she is watched, and is exasperated if she thinks anyone has noticed.

14

Pluto
(Saturn, Mercury, Earth)

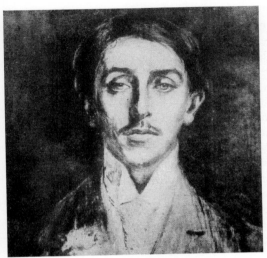

Maurice Barrès by J. E. Blanche

In his *Cratyle*, Plato writes: 'Hades (Pluto) is an accomplished sophist . . . his name may be derived from Aeides, the Invisible One; but more likely it was because of his capacity for knowing the value of things, that he was named thus.'

DESCRIPTION

The Plutonian shows a number of morphological features whose combination allows a precise description of the subject. Tall stature. A powerful head, with a severe expression and strong features. His face is: (i) very long, if Saturn predominates, (ii) full and square, if Earth predominates, (iii) anxious, if Mercury predominates. His hair is black and straight. His eyes are very dark and piercing, with flashes of light. His brow is wide and tormented. His nose is straight. His mouth and jaws are massive. His neck is quite short and strong. His shoulders are broad, his height above average.

The essential characteristic of the Plutonian is his sombre, grave expression and the dark piercing eyes which seem to scintillate powerfully. All his life-energy seems to be centred in his eyes. One is very aware of an individual who 'traverses vast immensities, veiled by darkness, and whose hold on life is derived almost entirely from the riches of the dead.'[1]

FUNCTION

Dominant faculty: sophisticated improvisation. Moral maladies: pride, envy, jealousy, avarice. Pluto has an 'inflexible heart'[2]. He is a despot who wants to rule over everything. Conquered by love, he surprises and brutally carries off the object of his wild passion.

Temperamentally violent, but taciturn, the Plutonian alternates moods of strange patience with terrible anger. Sometimes he is capable of any effort; at others, prone to total discouragement. He is two different men, the one robust and active, the other melancholic, weak and indolent. He can neither choose nor control his passions, which he usually tries to conceal. He is most often a poet who lacks the gift of form, who nonetheless dreams constantly of form, and may force himself to create it artificially for his own use. He is an artist who cannot express himself but creates bizarre designs; a seeker whose heavy hand fails to capture the delicate and shadowy thought that is incubating in the depths of his brain.

[1] Orpheus, *Hymn XVII*.
[2] Hesiod, *Theogony*.

149

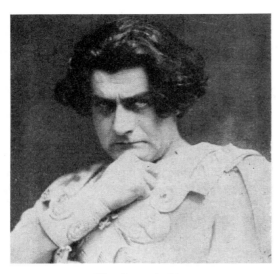

The Actor de Max

The Plutonian is a well-meaning cynic who was disappointed before ever experiencing his first true joy; he is inquisitive but never satisfied. He often hides an ardent soul behind a stony mask of sceptical and pessimistic serenity. This personality only appears in his unquiet, burning eyes.

Passionate by temperament, whole-hearted, a rigid philosopher, an ironic sophist, an implacable logician in his false reasoning, the Plutonian is usually solitary, distrusted and unhappy. He has a horror of solitude, which he is forced to seek through pride; the woman he loves often flees from him, or else, if not, he flees from her. She thinks him a tyrant and a despot, whereas he sees himself as the most timid and devoted of lovers.

He is a complex being who creates difficulties in his own life. He is proud, despotic and masterly, and at the same time timid and clumsy. He suffers in silence, for his proud despair would despise that which it adores. In secret he prostrates himself before the one whom he has made to suffer, and who rejects or despises him because of it. His anger and indignation can be terrible. In a fit of temper he knows no bounds. Insults pour out and the most unsuitable and even scatological expressions follow one another without regard to who may be listening, even if our Plutonian is supposed to be a gentleman. It is as if he were under the influence of some diabolical possession. In these circumstances he will be as vehement as at other times he is reserved and silent.

He is timid through arrogance and humble through pride. He prefers to take the last place if he has not been given the first. When he wants he can be brilliant and seductive, but as soon as anyone thinks they know him, he escapes. Inside he is a rebel. His mind is drawn to occult studies, to philosophy, to sophism, to contradiction, paradox and domination. His spirit moves through dark places, even though his intelligence may be brilliant.

THE PLUTONIAN WOMAN

The feminine type of Pluto is rare and may be classified as an aspect of the Mercury type. Saturn is very often missing, or else not apparent. She can be identified by her eyes, which are like black diamonds, and sparkle powerfully.

The Plutonian woman has a fiery temperament beneath a rigid and indifferent exterior. She never lets her guard be penetrated, so her sufferings are not known or even guessed at by others. She is a valiant woman, with qualities of energy and resistance, but nevertheless is usually awkward and misunderstood. She suffers in silence.

15

Proserpina
(Saturn, Venus, Earth, Luna)

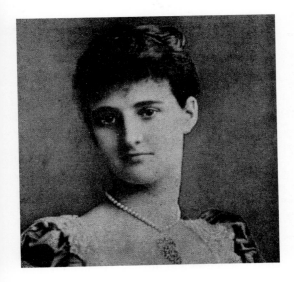

Proserpina, the daughter of Ceres, who was ravished by Pluto, is Queen of the Underworld. She spends only half of the year in her kingdom, and there exist sculptures of Mercury coming in Spring to fetch her, to restore vegetation to the earth.

DESCRIPTION

The Proserpina, or Persephone, type is always female, of medium or tall stature, depending on whether Earth or Saturn predominates. Her face is long and broad with a smooth complexion. The eyes are sparkling, black or blue. If Luna predominates they are blue; if Saturn, black. She has a Grecian nose, her mouth is full, with red lips. She has a firm chin.

Her waist is slim, supple and flexible. She has a narrow chest, with sloping shoulders but big thighs. Proserpina is a strong Mediterranean type, with the indolence of people born to live under a warm sun.

FUNCTION

Her character, like her temperament, is cool and yet sensual, tentative but lazy.

Proserpina women have an appetite for high living. They need worldly excitement, coupled with the comforts that millionaires can provide. Their dreams are of luxury and pleasure. Natural comediennes, they act out the comedy of existence with such astonishing naivety that it passes for a subtle form of flirtation. Flighty in appearance, but more faithful than she looks, jealous and very sensitive, Proserpina suffers from terrible depressions followed by manic euphoria. Like all those who combine contradictory types, some active and others passive, she is in danger of becoming melancholic if life keeps her away from the warm and sunny lands of which she dreams, even if she has never known them.

16

Neptune
(Saturn, Jupiter, Luna)

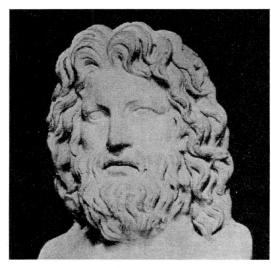

Neptune

The name of Poseidon (Neptune) is derived from *pollo eidos*: 'one who knows much'; and perhaps also from *o seion*: 'The Agitator[1].' This is how Plato explains it. The Neptunian learns easily, but this disturbs him, and he then disturbs others.

DESCRIPTION

Neptune is an impressive figure, combining the blue eyes of Luna, the high colour of Jupiter and the black hair of Saturn. Depending upon which of these is dominant – he is fairly tall, with strong limbs; he stands straight; his face is quite long; his expression is grave, with bold features, and always fresh complexion, azure blue eyes,[2] dark hair – and his energy is tempered with indolence. The Neptunian is proud

of his muscles and takes part in active sports, during which he no longer displays his customary indolence.

FUNCTION

His dominant faculty is imagination. His moral maladies include nervous debility and a tendency to drunkenness. The Neptunian is neither as old nor as frail as the Saturnian. His organism has more elasticity and a greater power of recovery. His character is less sombre and pessimistic, more fantastic, adventurous and sceptical. His blue eyes provide a glint of humour in his severe countenance. The thoughts of the Neptunian are a medley of poetry, idealism and dreams. His natural intuition leads him towards research that is both authentic and daring, as the combined influences of Jupiter and Luna give his temperament qualities of courage and vision denied to the Saturnian.

Sad and weary as Saturn, bold and noisy as Jupiter, crazy and restless as Luna, the Neptunian tends to instability insofar as the Saturn and Jupiter in him are in opposition and difficult to reconcile. The combination of these contradictory temperaments leads to physiological troubles and mental disharmony which should be foreseen, understood and exorcised. 'Boisterous Neptune' as described by Hesiod in *Theogony* may have strange impulses which distress his companions. Behind the appearance of vigorous health, the Neptunian conceals a temperament predisposed to circulatory and

[1] Plato, *Cratyle, Works T II*.
[2] Orpheus, *Hymn XVI*.

152

nervous disorders, and frequently suffers from attacks of chest pain that resemble angina pectoris. Sometimes Venus replaces Saturn in the Neptunian complex. The Venusian Neptune is self-centred, authoritarian and eccentric, voluptuous and neurotic.

To conclude, the Neptunian is authoritarian and eccentric, violent and capricious. He adds a lively, original wit to a robust appearance and an unstable nervous system. His interest is directed towards curiosities of all kinds, particularly among the natural sciences.

THE NEPTUNIAN WOMAN

The Neptunian woman is melancholy and strange, mysteriously seductive, though often unaware of it herself. She is Dido, Astarte, Salambo – to a Saturnian like Petrarch or Dante she could be Laura or Beatrice.

Queen or courtesan, hetaera or housewife, she is always distinguished, otherworldly, enigmatic. By nature haughty, she remains cold even whilst arousing passion. She seeks unusual sensations, and will not give herself to a man whom she can dominate – and therefore despise. She would be self-sufficient if she were not vain as well as cool; as an idol, she exacts her portion of incense or booty.

Nowadays the Neptunian often chooses to be a scientist. In an intellectual atmosphere she can realise her true gifts, and natural curiosity draws her towards the science of living things. Possessed of the aptitude to study life, she could become a doctor, with the certainty that she would never lack either coolness or perspi-

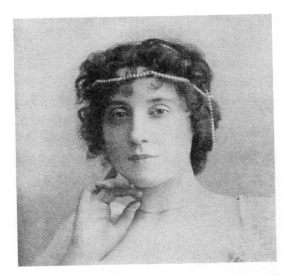

(photo Reutlinger)

cacity. She is not tender-hearted, her whims are deliberately planned, and she knows how to get exactly what she wants, gracefully.

Is she artistic? She should be a musician or a draughtswoman. As a musician she shows a talent for virtuosity; if she draws, she has a good sense for line, less for colour, and none at all for relief.

The less well-endowed Neptunian woman is mean-spirited. She is mocking and denigrating, envious and ironical. The Neptunian in his youth looks a little older than his actual age. At 25 he looks 30 or 35; he matures early, but then hardly changes at all, and remains vigorous for a long time; at about 45 he becomes fat and heavy. It is the same with the Neptunian woman – she is never young, but does not age.

17

Hebe
(Saturn, Luna, Apollo)

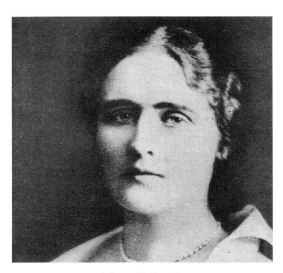

(photo Julietta)

Whether or not associated with other types, Hebe is always an immature, self-centred feminine type.

DESCRIPTION

Frail, girlish appearance. Her facial expression is placid and gracious, luminous but not sparkling. Long face. Regular features. Pale complexion. Light-coloured hair. Clear, beautiful, but expressionless eyes. Soft, flexible body.

Hebe has a beautiful supple body but lacks spirit. Her gestures are studied and artificial. She is pretty enough, but boring.

VARIATIONS

Hebe + Venus = Narcissus.
Hebe + Earth = Endymion, who only accepts the most discreet lovemaking, and indeed, sleeps through it.
Hebe + Mercury = Adonis.
Hebe + Mars = Hyacinth.
Hebe + Jupiter = Ganymede.

FUNCTION

The dominant quality is indifference. Moral malady: self-centredness. This may go to the length of suicide, in order to establish the desired image. A soft, vain, negative character, the lymphatic and very delicate Hebe is an inconstant, fickle type, given to coquetry and uninteresting frivolity.

18

Hercules
(Jupiter, Mars, with contributions from Earth, Luna and Venus)

'Hail, tyrant father, Hercules, with your heart full of courage,' says Orpheus[1], 'Hercules, whose enormous hands are endowed with prodigious strength, savage god of changing forms . . . powerful conqueror with massive limbs.'

The 'changing forms' of which Orpheus speaks are those which are derived from Earth, Luna or Venus. They are not essential elements of the Hercules type (Jupiter, Mars), but constitute additional possible types whose manifestations endow Hercules with a different character, according to which type is in the ascendant.

DESCRIPTION

A very muscular type, Hercules represents physical strength. He is a tall, well-built giant. Powerful head. His eyes are usually without lustre. A neck like a bull. Square, muscular shoulders.

FUNCTION

Dominant faculty: inventive intelligence. Moral malady: want of perseverance. Hercules represents powerful intelligence, not just muscular strength, capable of conceiving a gigantic plan of work and then executing it.

A type which combines Mars and Jupiter, Hercules may also derive something from Luna, Earth or Venus. These modify his behaviour and his temperament and give him either more fantasy, or more weight, or more intuition. He has the audacity and courage of a strong person, as well as the warlike attitude of a man who recognises no obstacles. But note that this strong man, this Samson, becomes as timid as an infant when it comes to dealing with feminine wiles or worldly astuteness. To please the whim of a courtesan he winds wool like a woman, while his enormous club is as useless as a baby's rattle. The hero who cut off the Hydra's heads and slew the vulture of Prometheus puts on the shirt of Dejanira; the conqueror of lions is poisoned by the fumes given off by the blood of a centaur. The psychology of the Herculean being is forever fixed by these legends. So too are the physiological and pathological disasters to which he most often falls victim, and for the same reasons – his strength, his courage and his excesses.

Generous and brave, although reckless and inconstant, Hercules has a mind which is powerful, thoughtful, even constructive, but is disconcertingly naive when tricked by cunning or obscured by passion.

---

[1] Orpheus, *Hymn XI*.

19

Juno
(Jupiter, Venus, Luna)

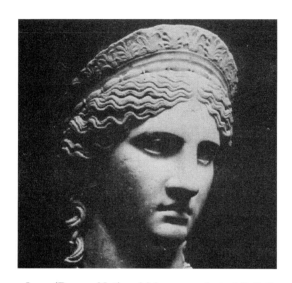

Juno (Rome, National Museum, photo Viollet)

Homer, in his 'Hymn to Apollo', describes Juno as 'feeling the rage of jealousy'.[1] She is typical of the shrewish, authoritarian, jealous wife and mother. Coming from the solid middle-class, she made a suitable marriage when she was very young; now she is constantly deceived, despite her indefatigable spying and her terrible jealousy.

DESCRIPTION

The metatype which results from this complex of Jupiter, Venus and Luna is exclusively feminine, handsome if a little heavy. As Hesiod put it, this terrible Juno 'of the alabaster arms', has a white body and plump flesh.[2] Her manner

[1] Homer, *Hymn* 'To Apollo'.
[2] Hesiod, *Theogony*.

is haughty, but in a vulgar way. Her gait is majestic. Her features are strong and regular, with an amber complexion and a fat face.

Her eyes are bright, sometimes cunning, sometimes hard. Valuable information may be gained from their colour:

Blue suggests there is fantasy in her despotism. She can take off, but will never fly too high.

Brown or gold shows a desire to dominate mentally. This Juno will seek a man whom she can push forward.

Black and sensual; she seeks to triumph by coquetry. Worldly or demi-mondaine, it does not matter, so long as she can reign and govern.

Black and dull shows a predisposition to hypochondria and neurosis.

Sparkling; beware of fits of temper which can lead to the worst excesses.

Her nose is aquiline, hooked or straight, and looks thin between her plump cheeks. Her mouth is a well-drawn bow with a disdainful fold. Her chin is either square – sign of an inflexible will, or round and fat – denoting obstinacy and a sensual appetite. Her well-built body is white, fat and fleshy. Her chest is opulent, her hips large. Her hands are shortish and heavy, often with spatulate fingers which belie her grand manner. She expresses herself in a loud voice, with vulgar gestures.

FUNCTION

Juno is a heavy, often lymphatic, woman. With advancing age her high colour and florid expression bestow a certain vulgarity, which may be further increased by drinking bouts, from which she hopes to gain energy. All that these do is augment her rages, by exasperating her already irascible humour.

Jupiter himself trembles before the rages of Juno, and he artfully seeks to appease the irritable mistress of his Olympian domain. He usually succeeds, for Juno is sensual. Despot against despot, it is the father of the gods who triumphs. He orders Mercury to put Argus to sleep, whilst he sets himself to flatter the instincts of his spouse. Juno forgives him and forgets her vengeance and jealousy, but begins to spy on him again the following day.

Dominant faculties: imagination, capriciousness. Moral maladies: authoritarianism and jealousy. Juno's character lacks harmony. Bad-tempered at home, she makes herself pleasant to strangers. Her masterful mind is superficial, and satisfied with second-best, and she dominates more through vehement language than by reason.

Haughty and authoritarian, imposing, demanding and jealous, she can be the masculine and headstrong woman who seeks to encroach upon the territory of men; you can sometimes see the suspicion of a beard on her chin. As a rival of man in her majestic beauty, Juno is as proud as the peacock, her special bird, and as boring as the rain, her special element. Fecund and monotonous, she maintains order in kingdoms and empires, and discipline in the home. Having chosen a weak husband, whom she overrules, she exercises her authority in bringing up her children.

20

Vulcan
(Mars, Venus, Mercury, Jupiter)

Hephaistos (Vulcan) is a son of Juno and Jupiter and brother to Mars and Hebe, but he does not resemble any of his family, nor indeed any of the other Olympian prototypes. It could be said that his physiognomy contributes a special prototype of its own, one which shatters the graceful harmony of Greco-Roman mythology by bringing in ugliness, infirmity, the club foot – the malignant dwarf, lame, despised, deformed and comical, and yet who incarnates the genius of industrial art.

He is a unipolar cerebral being who nevertheless became the husband of Venus. To understand him properly, study the myths which have been passed on by ancient poets:

Vulcan is the bearded hairy dwarf, a congenitally deformed being. Vulcan it was, feeble of body but powerful in mind, cerebrally virile, who inseminated inanimate matter and threw all the bitterness of his despair into the work. He took his revenge on humanity by creating Pandora, the courtesan decked out in the rarest jewels and endowed by Mercury and Minerva with every grace and every perversion, on the Titans by making Jupiter's thunderbolts, and on the Uranides when his Cyclopes forged the chains of Prometheus. He makes trinkets for the Nereids who flee from him, arms for the heroes who mock him, and gifts for the gods who despise him.

Vulcan creates ceaselessly, to distract himself, and for vengeance. He creates in order to forget his ugliness and for the feeling of power it gives him. He dreams of getting his mother under his control, perhaps in the hope of obtaining from her, through fear, the kisses denied to him from love or pity. He made for her a golden chair; anyone who sat on it could not rise unless he released them. Juno, unaware of the secret, admired it and sat on it. She was caught like a bird in a trap and Vulcan would not let her go. Mars, young, vigorous and ardent, ran to help his mother, easily fought off Vulcan, and rescued her. Vulcan then flew into a terrible rage, but as this had no effect upon the situation, he swore never to return to Olympus. Only Bacchus could coax him back, having first made him drunk. Drink could make Vulcan forget his resentment without affecting his mechanical genius. He hammered and spun the steel net in which Mars and Venus were trapped, so that the gods could laugh at their adultery (of which he was himself the victim), and he obliged Jupiter to return to him the dowry of his unfaithful spouse.

Hear what Homer causes him to say: 'You lucky immortals, gather round to see a funny sight! Because I am deformed, the daughter of Jupiter is always tormenting me with new outrages. At the moment she has attached herself to that pernicious Mars, because he is agile and handsome, whilst I am ugly and have twisted legs. My parents were entirely responsible for this misfortune, and should never have brought me into the world. The chains I forged for these two lovers will hold them until the day when Venus' father returns to me all the gifts I gave him in order to win his impudent daughter.'

Inventiveness is the weapon of this uncouth brother of Mars. He is ironical, like Mercury, and initiates a line that continues through Pan, the Satyrs, the Fauns and the Centaurs – a veritable series of monsters which introduces into its nomenclature the zoological characteristics favoured by the Egyptians.

158

DESCRIPTION

Vulcan is an exclusively masculine type. Thick black fuzzy hair, like a mane on his powerful head. A low broad forehead, lined by the constant effort to think. Black eyes sparkling with malice. A short hooked nose which wrinkles and bends. A big mouth whose corners are turned up in a sardonic grin, and whose commissures are deeply lined by bitterness. The chin juts forward, but is often hidden by a bushy black beard. The shoulders are massive, and curve like a dome over a small, thin, malformed body. The arms are thin but sinewy and terminate in vast bony hands. The legs are knock-kneed and of unequal length.

FUNCTION

Dominant faculty: creative imagination. Moral maladies: rebelliousness, anger, drunkenness. In spite of his debilitated and often rachitic constitution, Vulcan survives through intelligence and nervous energy. He has a sombre and passionate character, easily angered, always vindictive, never very good company, but his mental qualities and his remarkable inventive genius win him pardon for his violence and spite.

Brilliant and intuitive, independent and innovative, irrationally but powerfully creative, Vulcan is a tireless worker who only relaxes when he is drunk, not just in order to forget, but also to dream, and to recapture in his meditations the sarcastic philosophy that both avenges and upholds him.

21

Diana
(Mercury, Moon, Apollo)

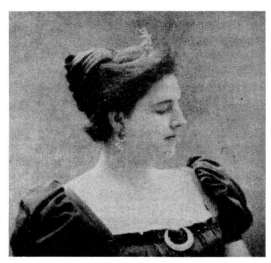

(photo Otto)

Diana Artemis is an androgynous type, feminine but with masculine tastes. She is Apollo's sister, and like him, an archer. She symbolises the independent woman, who is only interested in a man whom she can dominate.

The ancient hymn of Callimachus has it that the infant Diana, seated on the knees of Jupiter, addressed to him the following prayer: 'O my father, grant that your daughter may always remain a virgin, and bear as many names as Phoebus (Apollo). Give to me, as to him, a bow and arrows. Let me, too, carry torches and wear a fringed tunic that reaches to my knees and will not impede me from hunting. Give me as followers sixty daughters of Ocean who have barely reached puberty; and let eight other nymphs, whose duty it is to care for me whenever I am not hunting lynx and deer, look after my lace-up boots and my faithful hounds.'

Diana wants to equal her brother Apollo in strength, skill and agility, and to have the same privileges. She is a feminist. It is impossible for a man to please her and she would rather flirt with her nymphs. Actaeon surprised her whilst she was bathing naked; Diana changed him into a stag and he was devoured by his own hounds.

Listen to Orpheus: 'O Titaness amongst virgins, with the strong, hard heart . . . flirtatious huntress, pursuer by night. Many women are angry with you, a goddess who adopts masculine ways, incorruptible, wild . . . you will forever enjoy the springtime of life.[1] Yet you are the guardian of that most private part of woman . . . you are attractive to men . . . and you are unconquerable.'[2]

DESCRIPTION

Tall stature. Delicate features. Her face is a pure and graceful oval. Smooth pink complexion. Light brown hair, which is supple and fine. Her eyes are of a dark grey-blue colour, very beautiful but severe in expression, cold and hard as steel. Imperious gaze. Straight nose with narrow nostrils. Thin-lipped mouth, with a disdainful curve at the corners. Medium-sized, beautifully shaped ears. Graceful neck. Slim waist. Her limbs are slender but muscular. The legs are long in comparison with the trunk.

Diana is easily recognised by the steely blue eyes, the imperious nature of her cold, hard gaze, and the disdainful haughty expression of her lips.

[1] Orpheus, *Hymn XLVII.*
[2] Orpheus, *Hymn I.*

FUNCTION

Dominant qualities: coldness, intelligence. Moral maladies: pride, insensitivity, hardness. The muscular, haughty, authoritarian, egotistical type who is the Diana subject (and could be either a man or a woman) has a mind remarkable for its rapid grasp of ideas. Avid to learn, curious to know, but also capable of reflection, this individual is quick to make connections. Endowed with a strong power of assimilation, Diana is clever at transforming newly-received ideas into indisputable personal opinions. She is the patron of these women who have not yet given in to contact with or domination by men. She personifies a savage modesty. Remember that she caused Actaeon to be devoured by his own dogs for seeing her in the nude; yet she caresses Endymion because he remains asleep. She is a virgin, impulsive, proud and passionate, wild and independent. She is dedicated to all forms of sport and seeks to dominate both men and women.

VARIATIONS

Diana + Saturn = Proserpina.
Diana + Jupiter is to be found among the Muses.
Diana + Mars = Hecate. Her nostrils open almost vertically behind the tip of her aquiline nose, which is pointed like a bird's beak. She has red hair and a wilful, discontented expression, with green eyes full of spite and disdain.

'Pinched mouth, pointed nose. Better hang than meet with those.' is a popular saying about

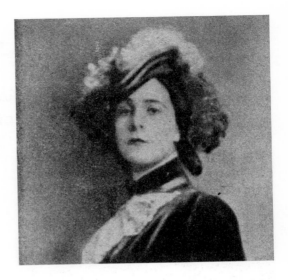

this bitter and peevish type. She is the Harpy, an infernal nymph who bristles with all the darts and plumes that she was able to tear from Love. But the true Diana is Mercury + Moon + Apollo, essentially cool and non-violent to all those around her. Diana lies in wait for her adversary and overcomes him at the very moment when he thought she was going to succumb to him. Consistent in the execution of her plans, she is inflexible both in defence and in the position she intends to hold.

The Lunar Diana is the true Diana, an unfeeling flirt – she does not give herself. She creates the impression of being a formidable enigma, apparently an idealist. In fact she is without ideals, but hides this behind an attitude which is at once both seductive and arrogant.

22

Bacchus
(Venus, Mercury, Terra)

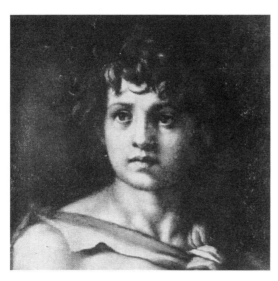

(Florence, Pitti Gallery, photo
Anderson-Giraudon)

Bacchus (or Dyonisos) is the spirit of Earth, as Ceres is its material substance. He is Wine to her Bread. Born of a thunderbolt from the thigh of Jupiter, the infant Bacchus is full of confidence, both in himself and in his power. Threatened with cerebral delirium and convulsions by a jealous divinity, he avoids madness by indulging in physical exercise. He hunts lions, tigers and lynx, then goes to sleep rolled up in a panther's skin, without worrying about anything; he feels free. But in adolescence he languishes. His graceful body is not very muscular, his chubby chest is almost feminine, and his limbs speak of indolence.

DESCRIPTION

The basic type of Bacchus may be Hermes (Mercury) or Aphrodite (Venus), associated with the vigorous and almost cubical body of Terra. He is both virile and feminine, with wide hips and breasts developed as in a woman, but with a man's face.

Tall stature, with a corpulent body, poor musculature, and a rounded outline. Slow, majestic walk. Beautiful black curly hair.[1] Open, laughing countenance.[2] Fresh complexion, eloquent eyes. Large, lined forehead, rectangular in shape – a 'bull's forehead'.[3] Black eyes, sparkling and mischievous. Aquiline nose, snub at the tip, with vibrant nostrils. Friendly, sensual mouth. Well-shaped, red, fleshy lips under a brown moustache. Wide hips and broad shoulders.[4]

With advancing age Bacchus becomes fat and vulgar, ill and often poor. He is tearful and desperate and his circumstances are tragic, but he consoles himself by getting drunk to forget the injustices and sorrows of his life.

FUNCTIONS

Dominant qualities: intelligence, charm and literary ability. Moral maladies: indolence, a tendency to drunkenness, and an exaggerated love of pleasure.

Jovial, audacious and enterprising, Bacchus is lord of the earth. 'He is the victor crowned with vine-leaves, who catches the moment as it flies.

[1] Orpheus, *Hymn XLVII*, Homer, *Hymn VI*.
[2] Orpheus, *Hymn XLVII*.
[3] Orpheus, *Hymn XXIX and XLIV*.
[4] Homer, *Hymn VI*.

He is king of the Present, who adapts everything to his needs. This god of the fleeting instant is as strong in his own way as Saturn, lord of enduring Time, but his strength is of a different kind; it bends and adapts itself to things, like the vine-stock among the stones. He follows the tide of life, and is adept at jumping higher for each return of the wave. He rises effortlessly in business, profession or politics.'[5] He is vigorous but indolent, an indolence which can be considerably ameliorated by physical exercise. He is extraverted, tough, inventive and brilliant, and prefers to juggle with ideas rather than to deepen them. His life is disorganised, consisting of an alternation of setbacks with lucky breaks. He is quick to master skills and could become famous through his grasp of reality and genius for adaptation.

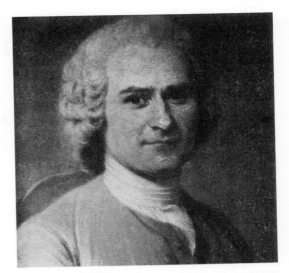

Jean-Jacques Rousseau, French School of XVIII century (photo Bulloz)

VARIATIONS

The Lunar Bacchus resembles Jupiter closely in appearance, character and temperament. The Marsian Bacchus is a faun, and can be recognised by his high, pointed ears. This type is very similar to Vulcan.

THE BACCHANTE

The female version of Bacchus is the Bacchante – a free-living girl who loves pleasure, movement, dancing, cheerful intoxication and an easy unrestricted life. Bacchantes may either give or sell their favours, depending on circumstances and the feeling of the moment. The Marsian Bacchante is the furious, cruel Maenad. The Lunar Bacchante resembles Proserpina. The Bacchante who is related to both the Moon and Mars is a variant of Hecate, the most terrible of them all. She is known as 'triple Hecate' – the Hecate of three heads: the head of a horse, Mars; the head of a jackal, Mercury; the head of a dog, Luna.

[5] Gary de Lacroze, *Les Hommes*.

23

Silenus
(Jupiter, Luna, Terra)

Silenus is an exclusively masculine type. In mythology there are two varieties of Silenus: one is short and squat, fat and vulgar; the other is tall, strong, muscular and attractive.

DESCRIPTION

Silenus, Short Type

Vulgar appearance. Big swollen nose with thick nostrils. Piggy little eyes in a florid red face. Big mouth with large red lips. Fat flaccid cheeks. Large, fleshy, low-slung ears. Very short neck. Squat obese body on short bowed legs.

His appearance is vulgar and common, his gestures gross, and he is often cheerfully noisy. His character is jovial and exuberant, he has a good solid constitution but is completely lacking in finesse. Short Silenus is the obtuse peasant, who is nonetheless capable of malice and guile.

Silenus, Tall Type

Tall stature. Calm, majestic appearance. Short square face. Straight or concave nose. Laughing blue eyes. Solid chin with powerful jaws. Thick neck. Strong shoulders.

Tall Silenus appears as a handsome giant with a strong, harmonious personality. Dominant quality: serenity. Moral malady: disdain, leading to distrust. Balanced and reserved, just and disinterested, tall Silenus is robust, equitable, observant and intuitive, and enjoys making syntheses.

He is a kind of Hercules, serene and likeable, strong enough to carry Bacchus, but too wise to wind wool at the feet of Omphale. In short, he is a sage who is capable of holding his liquor.

Pan
(Mercury, Mars, Venus, Saturn)

Exclusively masculine, Pan is of the same type as Vulcan but lacks the influence of Jupiter. He is the son of Mercury and a nymph, and is an artist and a craftsman. He lives among the Satyrs and the Fauns, who, like him, are nature-lovers, despite their sensual moods and savage bestiality.

DESCRIPTION

His long pointed face resembles that of a goat. Narrow, high tormented forehead. Bright greenish eyes with an oblique glance. High pointed ears. Well-developed chest. Broad shoulders and long arms. Narrow pelvis. Extraordinarily slender legs.

The appearance of his lower limbs has given Pan the name of 'goat-foot'. The Satyrs look even more like billygoats, but Pan is a goat-footed man, less lascivious and more capricious than the Satyrs.

FUNCTION

Dominant faculty: musical ability. Moral maladies: sensuality, lasciviousness. Flighty and capricious, Pan is a typical individualist and dreamer. He is a highly nervous person, eccentric, impulsive, inventive, argumentative and illogical.

Earth Types

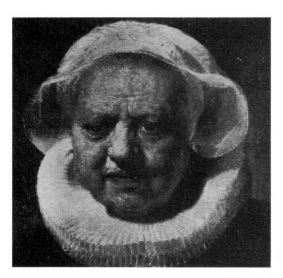

Rembrandt, *Portrait of an Old Woman* (National Gallery, photo Anderson Giraudon)

FLORA (Terra, Apollo)

An exclusively feminine type, the Flora woman is pretty and graceful, but soft. Her skin is smooth and white. Her face is well designed. Pink complexion. Bright, laughing luminous eyes. Straight nose. Sprightly expression.

These are delicate and pretty women. Pregnancy and childbirth are quite easy, but if Flora wants to suckle her child she becomes anaemic and debilitated and cannot easily regain her strength. Maternity causes her to lose her figure, but she nevertheless still manages to look pretty.

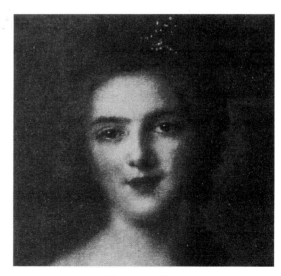

Metatype *Flora*
Nattier, *Madame Victoria* (Versailles Museum, photo Bulloz)

PURE EARTH (Gaia)

COMBINED TYPES

Flora   = Terra + Apollo
Rhea   = Terra + Mars + Saturn
Vesta   = Terra + Saturn + Apollo
Ceres   = Terra + Jupiter
Pomona   = Terra + Venus
Cybele   = Terra + Mercury
Proserpina = Terra + Saturn + Venus + Luna
            (see page 151)

RHEA (Terra, Mars, Saturn)

Rhea[1] is the girl who thrills to the sound of cymbals and tambourines, and the plaintive pipe[2] . . . Rhea, mastered in love by Saturn, brought into the light of day Vesta, Ceres, Juno, Pluto, Neptune and Jupiter.[3] She is the earth fortified, and is represented with a crown of turrets on her head.

Description

A bony, more or less emaciated body. Cubical head. Brown or reddish hair. Large forehead. The tip of her nose descends over her mouth. Tight lips. Fairly large ears. Jutting cheekbones.

The Earth+Mars type is always grumbling. He is taciturn, but shouts; ugly and unbearable, never laughs, and is very difficult to cheer up. The women often remain old maids.

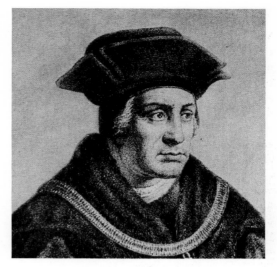

Thomas More (photo Cie des Arts Photomécaniques)

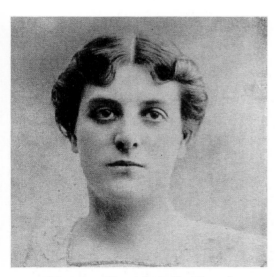

Metatype *Rhea* (photo Reutlinger)

[1] Orpheus, *Hymn XIII*, 'Parfum de Rhéa'.
[2] Homer, *Hymn XII*.
[3] Hesiod, *Theogony*.

VESTA (Terra, Saturn, Apollo)

Vesta is the Saturnian Earth, sad, mystical, essentially feminine, but chaste. She knows nothing of vile passion and has the aspirations of contemplatives, seers and saints. The most ancient of all types, 'Vesta, in the form of the divine Python, watches over the sacred temple of Apollo.'[1] Thus ancient lore justifies the composition of this metatype, Terra+Saturn+Apollo.

'The works of Venus do not please Vesta, the venerable virgin, firstborn of cunning Saturn, and the last to be released by him into the light of day on the order of great Jupiter. Touching the head of the powerful god of the shield, she took an oath to remain a virgin for ever.'[2]

Description
Long, wide face. Smooth, high, domed forehead. Dull brown eyes. Steep aquiline nose. Dainty mouth.

Functions
Dominant feature: somnabulism. Moral malady: melancholy.

Essentially feminine, but chaste, Vesta is predisposed to somnambulism, ecstasies and catalepsy, arising from the clash of her component types – heavy Earth, melancholy Saturn, frail Apollo. Her appetites and aspirations combine to form a mystical instinct, which she may encourage with the help of anaesthetic agents. She is a being who sleeps when she is awake, and watches in her sleep. Because it is impossible in our society to provide the modus vivendi for such a temperament, she is often charged with madness for what is quite simply the physiological behaviour of a special organism.

Vesta is in no way armed for the struggle of life. Goddess or saint, she is adored even as she is deplored. She may be an idol or a shadow, worth no more than her thoughts or her fantasies. She is a 'benevolent, dreaming, mystical, silent and reflective soul.'[3]

How can we preserve her? This depends upon circumstances, both her own and those of the environment in which she lives. Such women have precious qualities to offer, more than is usually imagined; but our civilisation neither appreciates nor understands them, for it does not know how to use them.

The Ancients looked after these women and regarded them as conscious sybils – Egerias who protected the state, apt as they were at all forms of divination. Moreover, this temperament can be modified by an appropriate lifestyle, with plenty of rest. To misunderstand Vesta is always either to sacrifice her or to submit to her.

[3] Homer, *Hymn XXIII.*

CERES (Terra, Jupiter)

An exclusively feminine type. Ceres, or Demeter, is the goddess of agriculture and harvest. 'Fair Ceres, her heart racked with sorrow . . .'[1] 'Isis, or in the language of the Greeks, Ceres.'[2] The statue of Isis is that of a woman with cow's horns, just as the Greeks represent Io.[3] 'Ceres, her beautiful blonde hair covered with an azure veil.'[4]

The name Demeter (Ceres) relates to the food she distributes, as a mother. Earth+Jupiter women appear in paintings of the Flemish school. They carry too much weight, and are undistinguished and excessively vulgar. They have light eyes and are very fertile.

[1] Homer, *Hymn IV.*
[2] Hesiod, *T II.*
[3] Homer, *Hymns IV and XII.* (In Egypt Isis was always veiled.)
[4] Plato, (Cratyle), *Works T II.*

[1] Homer, *Hymn XXIII.*
[2] Homer, *Hymn III* 'To Venus'.

POMONA (Terra, Venus)

A Mediterranean type. The eyes are more langorous, the nose less shapely, than in the pure Venus type. The nostrils vibrate. Pomona is superficial and not very intelligent. She has no depth, and for her, appearance is everything.

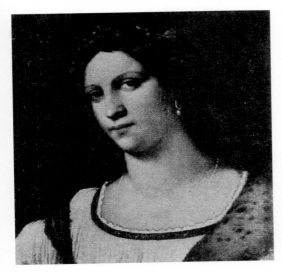

Metatype *Pomona*
Sebastiano dei Piombi, *La Fornarina* (Uffizzi Museum, photo Anderson-Giraudon)

CYBELE (Terra, Mercury)

Cybele is orientated towards material things and towards the man who provides them. She serves him, although not without deceit, moulding herself cheerfully to his tyrannical character. She is easily bogged down by detail. At whatever level of society, she serves, and cheats, and takes. At the bottom of the ladder she despoils her male victim on behalf of the strong man who looks after her interests. Scarcely less low, she cheats and lies to obtain gifts, and may then fall into the clutches of swindlers. Higher up, she makes herself indispensable to her provider. She is skilful and realistic. As a mother her servility becomes devotion, and she may even attain nobility of character.

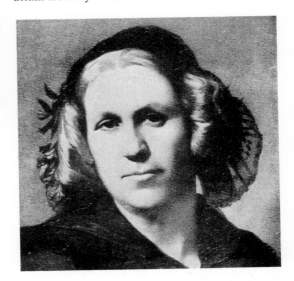

H. Flandrin, *Portrait de Madame Vinet* (Louvre Museum, photo Giraudon)

26

Reflections

Typology bears witness to Creation. Man is a created being, predisposed and predestined. Every human creature is a complex biological result of three formative forces: transmitted, acquired and potential.

The transmitted force, described by Paracelsus as the 'essence of the seed' – the natural pattern – is the result of legacies handed on by our forebears (atavism, heredity). The acquired elements which leave their mark upon the individual are of two main types: environmental, and pathological (disease). The potential, described by Paracelsus as the 'essence of becoming' is a pattern which contains all the properties or 'possibilities' characterising each individual, whose realisation would allow him to affirm his personality. The 'wholeness' of a person includes all the possibilities of action with which he has been endowed, and whose limits were decreed at his birth. This 'shape' of a person is significant – it expresses in signs the predisposition and predestination of an individual.

Hereditary predisposing factors confer a natural pattern that is manifested in the constitution. The constitution of a human being does not change, it remains 'that which is', the 'blueprint' for the development of an individual. Based on hereditary factors, a subject's constitution marks him from the time of his birth. There are three constitutions: Carbonic, Phosphoric and Fluoric. People of phosphoric constitution always have a tuberculous heredity, while Fluorics show signs of specific hereditary (syphilitic) disease, often going a long way back, and thus succeeding generations may be marked for a long time. This is of particular interest to the homoeopathic physician, as it enables him to read the signs and thus cure a number of disorders whose early origin is unknown, while at the same time assisting Nature to perform the transmutations necessary to ensure that the patient's descendants return to a normal state.[1]

The predestination of an individual may also be forecast. The study of a person's face yields exact signs whose interpretation bears on the behaviour of the subject, his intelligence, his character, his aptitude and his faculties. (Aptitudes relate to passive qualities, faculties are active.) 'Be what you are', Dr Henri Favre used to say, and then he would add, 'become what you can' – that is, what your potentiality will allow. Man is a created being who from the time of his birth has been endowed with a potential, and it is this potential he must use if he wishes to understand his destiny.

The destiny itself is not predetermined. It depends to a great extent on his own efforts, provided that they are directed and completed in harmony with his own unique natural possibilities. He must know what these are to develop them, and thereby realise his true worth. He should also be able to recognise them in other people, both for his own protection, and also so that he can help others to develop towards their own full potential.

Typology is a means of observing a human being, who bears within himself all the signs which allow us to discern his 'predispositions' and to foresee his 'predestination'. Careful study of an individual enables us to gather together the facts that concern his past, his

[1] Léon Vannier, *La Typologie et ses Applications Thérapeutiques*; Première Partie: Les Constitutions, 3rd edn (Doin, 1952).

170

present and his future. Although it is easy to 'look' at a human being, we have also to learn how to 'see' him. His signs are 'expressed'; it is for us to note, understand and interpret them.

The study of a subject's face and build provides details which will increase the accuracy of our diagnosis. Physiognomy enables us to make practical use of aptitudes, to train ability, and to encourage the realisation of values by conscious reflection.

Through typology we recognise the complex of possibilities presented by a human being. It is sufficient to identify the prototypes which can be seen in him. These are distinct, and by defining them we can demonstrate the real reasons for his failures or his lack of equilibrium.

The prototypes within a person may contradict one another or be discordant, resulting in internal tensions that upset the subject and those around him. Often, too, the faculties of one prototype have not been developed. A push in the right direction, at the right moment, from an informed observer, can bring new satisfaction into the life of that subject, revealing to him abilities of which he had previously been unaware.

Through typology we recognise the interior forces that characterise each human being. Of course, it must not be assumed that if only the whole of humanity was aware of its inner functions, there would be an increase of energies and perfect happiness all round. But it would be a first step in the right direction if each individual knew his potentialities – and his limitations – in which case he would undertake nothing that was truly beyond his capacity. Moreover, by applying his own insights to the people with whom he comes in contact, he would be better able to protect himself. This would be true self-defence and a powerful contribution to his survival.

The influence of the environment cannot be denied, but its importance should also not be exaggerated. 'Liberated from the maternal influence,' wrote Jacquin, 'the human being does not live only as the blind toy of passing forces. As a living unit of primordial quality, he paces his own vital rhythm to the rhythms that surround him, and consequently his form is shaped by those same influences.'[2]

Heredity and environment are not the only causes of our situation. Consider the definition of Paracelsus: 'An entity is the cause or the thing which is capable of directing the body.' We must understand this entity, this profound power within us, this mysterious force which animates us, this 'potential' which is not imposed upon us so much as 'given' to us, and which it is our duty to recognise fully.

At the same time, the individual is too often surrounded by hostile forces: unfavourable surroundings and provocative or deceitful companions who work against him. He feels bruised in his feelings and frustrated in his aspirations; disappointed by his own desperate and ineffective efforts, he cannot but be discouraged. His mood alters, his courage fails, his health declines and the signs of disease set in – not all illnesses are due to organic or microbial causes.

Indeed, the individual is very often not 'in order' – the order, that is, which corresponds to his constitution and type. Consider how many people practise a profession for which they are not only unprepared, but which is completely at odds with their aptitudes and faculties. Typology, by defining the 'virtual potential' of an individual, can bring powerful help in the mobilisation and direction of qualities previously unsuspected. The identification of these qualities is the aim of typological observation.

Can typology predict the future? No, but it can 'foresee' the development of the subject. If practised by an experienced and properly qualified person it can warn the subject against 'accidents' which might occur during the course of his life, whether moral, psychological, intellectual, physical, biological or pathological.

A human being is not the plaything of Fate. 'Every destiny can be planned,' affirmed the wise men of the Middle Ages. This planning is

---

[2] Jaquin, *L'Homme et les Hommes.*

most effective when the individual knows himself well, and can concentrate his will on delivering himself from the enemies within; when he restricts his ambitions to those that he can actually achieve; and when he is able to accept what was given to him at birth, and can bring himself to develop it, so as to realise to the full his own personality.

These ideas are important, insofar as they relate to the development of the individual, as well as to ensuring his physical and mental balance. There are many human beings who have not found their 'natural order', whose actions therefore do not correspond to their potential, and lead to disorders which affect their mental and physical status. In this alienation, whether deliberate or unconscious, the subject is working against his own nature and is no longer in rhythm with himself. He is 'dysrhythmic', ignoring the instructions with which he was originally provided.

No doubt the typologist, by imparting to the individual a knowledge of his own nature, can restore him to the order which he has abandoned – his own true order, which he may never have known. By revealing his dominant faculties, and putting him on guard against his besetting faults, he can save him from mistakes he might have made, and ensure him satisfactions which he might not have suspected. He can balance him, and to some extent 're-align' him, by describing the combination of types he possesses, whose elements can either form a benign association, or else clash dangerously. But the typologist's advice can only be effective if it is delivered to a subject whose informed will freely accepts the discipline. It is here that the physician can contribute powerfully, by giving the disorientated individual the balance he needs. Unfortunately, the physician has too often become a monstrosity whose destructive activities, scientifically supported by infallible doctrines, will soon result in the disintegration of both patients and doctors. Patients, gathered in flocks parked in multiple administrative sectors, must undergo the judgement of their doctors, it being understood that both will be deprived of all freedom, their reasons for being treated and for treating to be dictated by an absolute authority. It is true that there are doctors who wish to remain 'free', but their protestations are unheeded. Technical excellence overshadows clinical acumen. The findings of laboratories and specialists, entrenched in their watertight compartments, are sufficient to establish a 'scientifically controlled' diagnosis in which the patient, a created human being, is not only abandoned but completely ignored.

A reaction is beginning to appear. 'How can the medical technician know what the patient *has* if he does not know what he *is*?' writes Gustave Thibon.[3] The question is admirably put. How can it be answered if the doctor is unaware of typology? Consider the words of Claude Bernard: 'A doctor is the doctor, not of the human race at large, but of one individual in circumstances of illness peculiar to himself.' It has been said often enough that there are no diseases, only sick people – 'It is I who am ill,' writes Thibon. 'I have a heredity, a temperament and a character which belong to no one but me. I have also a family, a profession and a circle of friends, and my illness, in a way, partakes of all this.'

Homoeopathy is that form of medicine which can be adapted to the human being, since its remedies are indicated by the symptoms which express the patient's personal reactions. These symptoms must not be considered only as the means of making a clinical diagnosis. All the signs that the subject presents are important, whether they are objective or subjective, neurological or functional, physical or psychological. All express an attitude to life and all can be matched to the characteristics of homoeopathic remedies.

There are no imaginary invalids. It is not helpful for a homoeopath to refer for psychoanalysis a 'sad person' who is debilitated, 'indifferent to everything, to his own affairs,

---

[3] *Qu'Attendez vous du Médecin?*, Présences (Plon, 1953).

and even to his family', who is 'irritable with others and with himself', 'seeks solitude' and 'shuns society.'[4] The indications for Sepia are obvious, but it is also useful to know whether the subject has Saturnian qualities, in which case one can warn him against the exaggeration of his type.

An informed typologist will know the principal remedies for the prototype under consideration; the homoeopath can give an exact prescription for an acute or a chronic condition. He knows how to evaluate the signs shown by the subject, under the headings of Typological, Clinical and Therapeutic. The healthy subject, the sick subject and the remedy must not be dissociated in our minds. A knowledge of the healthy subject is necessary so that changes can be judiciously noted, and indeed foreseen. A deep knowledge of the sick person is indispensable, since illness, even acute illness, is not spontaneous – it always has a cause. Identification of the true cause of the pathology observed is essential if the individual is to be properly treated.

The modern physician is regarded as a competent scientist who examines patients and makes diagnoses. The homoeopath is a prudent observer who understands the patient, seeking for the causes, whether intrinsic or extrinsic, which underlie his human functions and their pathological changes. The well-chosen remedy acts as a mediator between the subject as he is found, and as he was before he was changed by illness. The safe, infinitesimal dose will rapidly restore the patient to his normal condition, that is, to the state which corresponds to his personal function as defined by analysing the types which constitute him. Jean Koller wrote, 'Authentic health is directed by the Spirit.' Homoeopathy is not the whole of medicine, but an important part of it – perhaps the most important. It is the 'human medicine' demanded by patients who have grown tired of being deceived and abused.

---

[4] The words between quotation marks are the characteristics of Sepia, extracted from the homoeopathic materia medica.

27

Conclusion

Due credit must be given to those Masters who, in their writings, preached medicine on the human scale, even though they were unable to bring it into being. The secret is expressed in a few words: 'Exact knowledge of the human Being' and 'faithful obedience to, and respect for, his Creator.'

It must be said that in this day medicine lacks virtue. The word is used deliberately – virtue, from the Latin *virtus*, means power, the vital force which resides in every man. It has nothing to do with respectability, which is an assumption of dignity and piety inspired by the fear of criticism. It is something much greater than this. The physician's virtue is an immanent force which enables him to fulfil his vocation. It speaks of a higher power, substantial as well as spiritual, whose many aspects uplift and fortify his mind: nobility of character, independence, purity of heart, lucid thinking, a strong will, firmness, insight, perception, benevolence, goodness, honesty, sincerity, disinterestedness, modesty. This 'virtue', which is the hallmark of the true healer, cannot be learned from textbooks.

The physician must be *both the servant and the minister of Nature*. Hippocrates and Paracelsus are agreed on this point. But how is the physician to know Nature if he has not learned about her, for his whole education is directed away from such ideas. As for the human being, with his uniquely human behaviour – what will become of this in the litany of facts and tests which constitute the student's only learned knowledge? The virtue of a physician is powerless when it is based on a desperate ignorance of the subject whom it is supposed to help. The virtue of a physician fails when it lacks the means to *see*, to *understand*, to *treat* and to *heal*.

It is not always easy to write a homoeopathic prescription, and often, after the consultation and when he has had time to study the patient's notes, the homoeopath finds that he has to alter it. But how rewarding it is to see the patient recover in a few months from a complaint he may have endured for years. If the physician is old he will know several generations of a family; he can follow the evolution of temperaments and assist the parents to a better understanding of their children. He can attract the attention of the young, by showing them what they are and what they could be. In using his beneficent influence he will encourage them to undertake the projects for which they are potentially suitable. He is the true family physician, the one who is consulted, not only for physical disorders, but also for emotional and moral problems.

No matter what dramas humanity plays out before him, the physician may not be proud, or vain of his reputation, since he is constantly aware of one of the anxieties connected with his profession – the fear of making a mistake. His responsibility grows with his knowledge, and if to err is human, then he must not expect to be right every time. Let it just be said that he will do his best, and that his best will be very good if he remains a faithful observer, and if he reflects upon the fact that what he knows has not been given to him, so much as entrusted to him.

Paracelsus stated that the art of the true physician is a gift emanating from God. We take leave to add: true art does not seek the cause of that which is, but rather the *infinite potential*.

Adamantius, *Treatise on Physiognomy* (1760).

Agrippa, *Occult Philosophy or Magic* (1727).

Allendy, *Les Tempéraments* (1920).

Anonymous, *Letters on Physiognomy* (1801).

Arone, *La Morphologie Humaine* (1915).

Belliere, de la, *Physionomia Rationalis* (1666).

Belot, *Oeuvres* (1672).

Bessonnet-Favre, *La Typologie* (1910).

Bessonnet-Favre, Manuscript notes.

Binet, *Morphologie Médico-artistique de la Femme*.

Blondel, Maurice, *L'Etre et les Etres* (1935).

Bouchet, *La Cosmogonie Humaine* (1917).

Bruyères, *La Phrénologie, le Geste et la Physionomie* (1847).

Cardan, *La Métascopie* (1658).

— *De la Subtilité* (1642).

Chaillou and MacAuliffe, *Morphologie Médicale (1911)*.

Commelin, *Mythologie Grecque et Romaine* (1909).

Corman, *La Constitution Physique des Paralytiques Généraux* (1932).

— *Visages et Caractères* (1932).

— *Quinze Leçons de Morpho-psychologie* (1937).

Crollius, *Basilica Chymica* (1608).

Favre, *La Série Humaine* (1856).

Gary de Lacroze, *Les Hommes* (1890).

Guenot, *La Genèse des Espèces Animales* (1932).

Helvetius, *Microscopium Physiognomia Medicum* (1576).

Hesiod, *Theogony*, trans. Mazon (1928).

Hippocrates, *Complete Works*, trans. Littré (1841).

Homer, *Hymns*.

Jacquin-Chatellier, *L'Homme et les Hommes* (1932).

Johannes-Valentin, *De Varietate Facies Humanae* (1676).

Kretschmer, *Body Structure and Character* (1930).

Lavater, *La Connaissance de l'Homme* (1806).

Leclerc, *La Physionomie*.

Lecomte de Nouy, *L'Avenir de l'Esprit* (1941).

Ledos, *Traité de Physionomie Humaine*.

Lenclos, *L'Etude Objective des Tempéraments* (1932).

MacAuliffe, *Development, Growth* (1923).

Melampus, *Divination by the Natural Markings of the Body*, addressed to King Ptolemy.

Ménard, *La Mythologie dans l'Art Ancien et Moderne* (1878).

Metososiasia, Italian Manuscript.

Nicolle, *La Destinée Humaine* (1936).

Osmond, *Traité de Physiognomie* (1946).

Paracelsus, *Complete Works* (1658).

Péladan, *L'Art de Choisir sa Femme* (1903).

— *Comment on Devient Artiste* (1894).

— *Sciences Occultes* (1908).

— *La Dernière Leçon de Léonard de Vinci* (1909).

— *De l'Androgyne* (1910).

Plane, *La Physiologie, ou l'Art de Connaître les Hommes* (1797).

Polti and Gary, *La Théorie des Tempéraments* (1847).

Porta, *La Fisionomia del Uomo* (1652).

Ribot, *La Psychologie des Sentiments*.

Richer, *Introduction à l'Etude de la Figure Humaine*.

— *Morphologie de la Femme* (1920).

Robert, *Nouvel Essai sur la Mégalantropogénésie* (1803).

Roy, *Traité du Rire* (1814).

Schmitt, 'Du Retour Permanent à la Constitution Primitive'. *Homoeopathie Française* (February 1951).

Schneider, *Human Types* (1937).

Sedir, *Les Tempéraments et la Culture Psychique, d'après Jacob Boehme* (1894).

Stratz, *La Beauté de la Femme*.

Sue, *Essai sur la Physionomie des Corps Vivants Considérés depuis l'Homme jusqu'à la Plante* (1797).

Thooris, *La Médecine Morphologique*.

Vannier, Léon, *L'Homoeopathie Française* (articles since 1912).

— *Homoeopathie, Médecine Française* (1949).

— *Conférences au Centre Homoeopathique de France* (1951, 1952, 1953).

Vialleton, *L'Origine des Etres Vivants* (1929).

Voenio, *Tractatus Physiologicus de Pulchritudinae* (1797).

Zahn, *Liber Admirabilis Oeconomi Mundi* (1646).

Aconite, **99**, 100, 101, 104
Actaea Racemosa, 81
Aesculus, **101–2**, 104
Aloes, 101, **102**, 104
Anacardium, **28**, 29, 31, 63, 80
Antimonium Crudum, 128, **130–1**, 132, 133
Argentum Nitricum, 114, **115**, 119
Arsenicum Album, **65–6** 67, 69, 102, 104, **114**, 115, 119
Aurum Metallicum, **28–9**, 31, 46

Baryta Carbonica, 46, 49, 142, 144
Belladonna, 84
Berberis, 46, 49
Borax, 84
Bryonia, **99–100**, 104

Calcarea Carbonica, 2, **79–81**, 82, 84, 85, 87
Calcarea Fluorica, 2, 80
Calcarea Phosphorica, 2, 68, 82
Causticum, 46, 49
Chamomilla, **28**, 29, 31, **116–17**, 119
Colocynthis, **28**, ʼ29, 31

Dulcamara, **131–2**, 133

Ferrum Metallicum, **64**, 66, 69, 84

Gelsemium, **28**, 29, 31, 46
Graphites, 79, **85**, 87, 103

Helonias, 85
Hepar Sulphuris, 99, **100**, 104, 142, 144
Hydrastis, 85, 87

Ignatia, **67–8**, 69, **117**, 119, **131**, 133
Iodum, **64–5**, 66, 69, **114–15**, 119
Ipecacuanha, 84

Kali Carbonicum, **64**, 65, 66, 69

Lachesis, 86, **116**, 119

Lilium Tigrinum, **116**, 119
Lycopodium, 25, **26–7**, 31, 101, 104, 141, **142**, 144

Medorrhinum, 49, 85, 87, 117, 119
Millefolium, 84
Natrum Muriaticum, **62–3**, 64, 66, 68, 69
Natrum Sulphuricum, 46, 85, 87, **128–30**, 131, 133
Nux Moschata, 131, 133
Nux Vomica, **27–8**, 29, 31, 46, 49, 82, 84, **100–1**, 104, **141**, 142, 144

Opium, 142, 143, 144

Phosphorus, **66–7**, 69, 102, 104
Platina, 83
Plumbum Metallicum, 46
Psorinum, 49, 103, 104, 117, 119, 144
Pulsatilla, **67**, 68, 69, 84, 85, 87, 102, 103, 104, 128, **130**, 131, 133

Rhododendron, **131**, 133
Rhus Toxicodendron, 46, 83, 129, **131**, 133

Sabina, 84
Secale, 83
Sepia, **45**, 46, 49, 83, 84, **141–2**, 144
Silicea, 81, 82, **113–14**, 119
Solidago Virga, 46, 49
Spiritus Quercus Glandium, **29**
Stannum, 67
Staphysagria, **29**, 86
Sulphur, **25–6**, 27, 31, 49, **98–9**, 100, 102, 103, 104, 141, 142, 144
Sulphur Iodatum, 100
Syphilinum, 49

Thlaspi Bursa Pastoris, 84
Thuja, **45–6**, 49, 79, 85, **86**, 87, 131, **132**, 133
Trillium Pendulum, 84
Tuberculinum, 49, 69, 100, 104, 117, 119

CLASSICAL HOMOEOPATHY

Dr Margery Blackie
Edited by Dr Charles Elliott and
  Dr Frank Johnson
360 pages, 216 x 138 mm, 1986, Repertory Edition
1990, ISBN 0906584140

This book sets before the reader the enthusiasm, learning and deep clinical understanding of one of the foremost homoeopaths of our time.

Classical Homoeopathy draws into one volume Dr Blackie's teaching over the whole span of her career. The first part describes the thinking behind homoeopathy and the principles on which the successful homoeopathic prescription is based, with its recognition of the sick person as a body, mind and spirit relationship, bound inseparably as one. The major constitutional remedies are then studied in detail, either individually or differentiated within groups of related remedies. This is followed by the symptomatic treatment of illness or disability, analysing each of the remedies that may be of value, and distinguishing the particular circumstances in which one remedy is likely to be indicated in preference to another. Next there is a compact materia medica, summarising the essential characteristics of one hundred and eleven major remedies. The final part comprises a clinical repertory, relating symptoms to remedies already discussed in the book, and an index of remedies.

'It is an essential book for all those with a genuine interest and belief in homoeopathy, for it reveals so clearly Dr Blackie's incomparable style of practice and knowledge of materia medica. However, the complete beginner will be swamped with so much fact, and would be wise to delay purchase for a short time until they have gained a working knowledge of homoeopathy. Thereafter, the book will be invaluable.'   *Homoeopathy*

EVERYDAY HOMOEOPATHY

Dr David Gemmell
184 pages, 216 x 138 mm, 1987,
ISBN 0906584183

This book shows you how to use homoeopathic medicine in the everyday context of your own personal and family health care. It covers the problems that the lay person is quite likely to have to cope with, either as first aid or else in a wide variety of complaints and disorders that may not be urgent but where relief and cure are sought.

The author starts by describing the thinking behind homoeopathy, its stress on the need to assess the patient in his or her entirety as an individual, and its freedom from toxic side-effects. There is the necessary basic information on how to observe symptoms and select a remedy, as well as on potency and dosage.

The main part of the book is presented in four sections – accidents and first aid, the problems of women, children's problems and general problems. The author explains the nature of each problem and suggests common-sense measures to be taken whatever else is done. He then discusses the various personal circumstances and particular symptoms that may be present, using these to point to the appropriate homoeopathic self-treatment.

He highlights the cases where self-help is out of place and medical advice must be sought without delay. He also highlights the cases where homoeopathy can provide a more complete and effective cure, but where self-help is equally inappropriate and a professional homoeopathic evaluation must be obtained.

'For years now my patients have been asking me what the best book is to help them understand how they can use homoeopathy for their family. I have always been uneasy about the books I've had to recommend because they always seem to fall short of the ideal. . . . At last someone has written this book, and it comes across as the work of a thorough, caring, down-to-earth physician who knows just what he is talking about.'   *Holistic Health*

HOMOEOPATHIC PRESCRIBING

Dr Noel Pratt
87 pages, 216 x 120 mm, revised edition 1985,
ISBN 0906584035

This book is written for all who use homoeopathic remedies. Clear indications are given wherever it is important that the lay person should also obtain medical advice.

One hundred and fifty-six common complaints and disorders are covered in the book, arranged alphabetically. A selection of appropriate remedies is then listed, together with details of the particular symptoms and signs that enable the prescriber to differentiate between each of them. There is an appendix on the constitutional types. The book is printed with interleaved blank pages, to enable the reader to amplify the text on the basis of personal experience.

'Dr Pratt has written a very useful vademecum for those with a good working knowledge of homoeopathy. The way the book is set out makes for clarity and ease of access to the appropriate information.'

Homoeopathy Today (UK)

HOMOEOPATHY AS ART AND SCIENCE

Dr Elizabeth Wright Hubbard
Edited by Dr Maesimund B. Panos and
  Della DesRosiers
344 pages, 216x138 mm, 1990,
ISBN 0906584264

Dr Elizabeth Wright Hubbard was one of the most brilliant homoeopaths of the twentieth century. This book represents a large part of her teaching and writing, setting before the reader her great gift of being able to describe homoeopathy in a way that imprinted itself in the minds of all who studied with her.

She begins by examining the nature and philosophy of homoeopathy and its relationship with conventional medicine. This is followed by a discussion on the use of the repertory and then by a major section on remedies, in which she displays her wide-ranging and often intuitive mastery of the materia medica. There is a further major section on cases, demonstrating the skill with which she was able to match the symptom picture of the patient to the proved indications of the relevant remedy. The final section of the book comprises the famous 'Brief Study Course in Homoeopathy'. Here she explains in expanded

detail how the homoeopath proceeds in the evaluation and management of the individual case.

'What a treasure trove this book is, a posthumous collection of essays from one of the most brilliant homeopaths of the twentieth century. . . . They are perhaps the most pleasurable way for someone schooled in allopathic thinking to grasp the essence of the homeopathic mind. They illustrate the idea of the simillimum, the minimum dose, and the single remedy in a way which mentioning these principles here does nothing to convey. . . . They are essentially anecdotal evidence and they are essential reading. When the inadmissible evidence has been disclosed we have learned the truth.'

Homeopathy Today (USA)

HOMOEOPATHY IN PRACTICE

Dr Douglas Borland
Edited by Dr Kathleen Priestman
208 pages, 216x138 mm, 1982, Symptom Index
Edition 1988, ISBN 090658406X

Dr Borland presented this material as a course during the 1930s at the London Homoeopathic Hospital. His homoeopathic insight remains as fresh and as valuable today as it ever was.

The book is divided into two sections. The first, entitled 'Homoeopathy in Clinical Conditions' deals in turn with injuries and emergencies (including acute pain), headaches, sore throats, respiratory and heart conditions, obstetrics and gynaecological conditions, sleeplessness, and pre- and post-operative conditions. The second section, 'Studies and Comparisons of Remedies', shows to what extent Dr Borland excelled in the way he led from one remedy to another, often linking them by their differences or similarities. He first looks at six Kali salts, and then at five Natrum salts, all well known to the homoeopathic prescriber. 'Seventeen Important Remedies' are then discussed, and a comparison made between three more – Lilium Tig., Natrum Mur. and Sepia. The final chapter deals with the use of four nosodes – Psorinum, Tuberculum Bovinum, Medorrhinum and Syphilinum. A remedy index and a symptom index complete the work.

'The book comprises some fourteen chapters, nine devoted to a study of various clinical conditions, and five to studies and comparisons of remedies. Even when the conditions are common and we all have to deal with them daily, the treatment is fresh and there are unusual angles on well known remedies and interesting comparisons on smaller remedies.'

The Homoeopath

INSIGHTS INTO HOMOEOPATHY

Dr Frank Bodman
Edited by Dr Anita Davies and Dr Robin Pinsent
119 pages, 216 x 138 mm, 1990,
ISBN 0906584280

The purpose of this book is to show that it is possible to subject homoeopathy to the same standards of intellectual scrutiny that apply to any other branch of medicine.

The author begins by explaining this specialty as it first confronts the conventionally-trained mind, and follows with an analysis of the extraordinary contribution made by its founder, Dr Samuel Hahnemann, to modern medicine. There are several chapters on the use of homoeopathy in psychiatry, in which Dr Bodman had much experience. He then discusses the homoeopathic management of a wide variety of clinical conditions, including allergy – the area where research during the 1980s has demonstrated the effectiveness of the microdose. He concludes with a discussion of the reasoning that lies behind research into homoeopathy.

'The possibility of achieving a lasting cure is squarely counterpoised to the palliative aim of much orthodox drugging . . . . It is clear that the author has not just read, but studied and considered carefully the meaning of Hahnemann's writings.' *The Homoeopath*

INTRODUCTION TO HOMOEOPATHIC MEDICINE, Second Edition

Dr Hamish Boyd FRCP
285 pages, 216 x 138 mm, 1989,
ISBN 0906584213

This book provides a systematic introduction to the principles of homoeopathic medicine. It shows how the homoeopath's selection of a remedy is based on a process that goes beyond the diagnosis of a particular condition to a perception of the patient as a whole and individual person.

The homoeopathic materia medica is discussed in relation to the systems of the body and the patient's presenting complaints, in a framework that will be familiar to any doctor. The author uses this framework to describe the subsequent management of the patient in homoeopathic terms. He describes the clinical conditions in which homoeopathy is particularly useful, and those where conventional treatment is likely to be necessary, as well as the circumstances where orthodox medicine and homoeopathic medicine can fruitfully be used in conjunction with one another.

The symptom pictures of fifty-five of the most important remedies are then described in detail, offering the reader a sufficient basis on which to introduce them into his or her own practice. Dr Margaret Tyler's valuable 'Study of Kent's *Repertory*' is given as an Appendix.

'The book is clearly laid out and well presented. The material is divided into clearly defined chapters which make it easy to dip into. I felt it succeeds well as an introduction to homoeopathic medicine, presenting the material simply, but at the same time leaving nothing out. I liked particularly the way in which Dr Boyd expressed the importance of utilising the best of homoeopathic medicine and the best of orthodox medicine. He got the balance just right.' *The Homoeopath*

MATERIA MEDICA OF NEW HOMOEOPATHIC REMEDIES

Dr O. A. Julian
637 pages, 216 x 138 mm, 1979, ISBN 0906584116

This book offers a rich collection of over a hundred new homoeopathic remedies. It adds to existing knowledge, supplementing the classic materia medicas. Some of the remedies are completely new. Others are familiar substances used homoeopathically for the first time. Most of them have been the subject of a Hahnemannian proving, while the remainder have undergone a clinical symptomatological study and their value has been confirmed in therapeutic use.

A detailed clinical repertory is provided at the end of the book, together with an index of clinical keynotes. Principal symptoms are italicised throughout the text. There is a bibliography for each remedy, as well as chemical information of pharmaceutical relevance.

'Dr Julian must be complimented on beginning the reappraisal of the existing materia medica for the late twentieth century, and for introducing in critical fashion so many new remedies.' *Homoeopathy*

STUDIES OF HOMOEOPATHIC REMEDIES

Dr Douglas Gibson FRCP
Edited by Dr Marianne Harling and
  Dr Brian Kaplan
538 pages, 216 x138 mm, 1987,
ISBN 0906584175

Homoeopathic remedies come from every part of the world and from all the kingdoms of nature – mineral, vegetable, animal and microbe. They include strong poisons such as arsenic, the venom of deadly snakes and the products of disease, as well as harmless substances like sand and charcoal, and herbs whose healing properties have been handed down through generations and are celebrated in history and legend.

Dr Douglas Gibson was a distinguished homoeopath who recognised the importance of knowing the materia medica in depth. These studies of remedies, first published in the British Homoeopathic Journal over the period 1963– 1977, combine the panorama of each remedy with a faithful description of the mental and physical symptoms it elicits from a sensitive prover. The whole remedy is indeed used to treat the whole patient.

His studies are edited here for publication in book form. They differ from any previously published materia medica in the uniquely wide range of insights that are brought to bear on each remedy. They will be of great practical value, and a source of pleasure and stimulation, to the homoeopathic clinician.

'This is a classic text in which author, editors and publishers have proved equally worthy of each other. It will assist the neophyte and established homoeopath equally in becoming more competent and reliable prescribers.'
British Homoeopathic Journal

TUTORIALS ON HOMOEOPATHY

Dr Donald Foubister
200 pages, 216 x138 mm, 1989,
ISBN 0906584256

This book offers the reader an insight into Dr Foubister's clinical experience, gained over a long career in homoeopathic practice. His writings are remarkable for the extent of his knowledge and his close attention to detail.

The contents reflect many of his particular strengths. The first section studies the factors that underlie the homoeopath's evaluation of the individual patient. This is followed by a section of several chapters on paediatrics, in which he excelled. There is then a comprehensive section on Carcinosin – his development of the Carcinosin remedy picture was his major contribution to homoeopathy and it gained him worldwide acclaim. He then discusses a number of other remedies in detail, with a final section on specific conditions. The book ends with an Appendix of therapeutic hints that had served him well.

'Dr Foubister has managed in masterly fashion to compress his immense knowledge of virtually the whole field of this fascinating discipline, encompassing his life experience in clinical research with special reference to his own particular expertise in paediatrics.'
Homoeopathy Today (UK)

HERBAL MEDICINE
Dr R.F. Weiss
Translated from the 6th German edition by
A. R. Meuss. 362 pages, 246 x 189 mm, 1988,
ISBN 0906584191

Herbal Medicine is the English translation of the current Sixth Edition of *Lehrbuch der Phytotherapie*, a book which has established itself as an indispensable modern text in the field of medical herbalism. This latest edition takes full account of present-day research findings, from which Dr Weiss has added many further suggestions for prescriptions, as well as indications for new areas of application.

The introductory chapters examine the nature of the subject and provide the necessary guidelines for prescribing. The main part of the book then studies the large and impressive body of plant drugs, arranged on a basis of clinical diagnoses relating to particular systems – digestive, cardiovascular, respiratory, urinary, nervous, female reproductive, the skin and the eyes. There are separate chapters on influenza and colds, rheumatic conditions, some metabolic and endocrinal disorders, the use of herbal medicine in cancer, the treatment of wounds and other injuries, and the therapeutic use of herbal baths.

In every case the relevant plants are discussed, with information on their occurrence and botanical features, differentiation from related species, constituents and medicinal actions. Many of them are illustrated by line diagrams. The treatment sections offer a wealth of suggested prescriptions, with details of dosage, application and precautions. Where appropriate, proprietary formulations are also included. Full references are given throughout. There is a comprehensive subject index of almost two thousand entries.

'It is refreshing to have in English an established practical work from the hands of a senior medical practitioner who has used herbal remedies for over six decades. . . . The strength of this book is in its appearing like a written account of an apprenticeship with a master craftsman: that alone will make it compulsory reading for anyone interested in using herbal remedies well.'

Complementary Medical Research